women without sex

the truth about female impotence and other sexual problems

CATHERINE KALAMIS

SELF-HELP DIRECT

For more copies of this book, please send £10.95
cheque or postal order per book
(overseas sales $25 per book, postage & packing
free) made payable to *Self-Help Direct* to:
Self-Help Direct Publishing
PO BOX 9035,
London, N12 8ED

DESIGN: Michael Crozier/Design Unlimited
COVER ILLUSTRATION: Michael Daley
GRAPHICS/ILLUSTRATIONS: Michael Roscoe

Published by Self-Help Direct Publishing, PO Box, London, N12 8ED
First edition 1999

ISBN 1 900461 25 0

contents

Introduction

Sex . . . 'it's half of where your feelings come from. I would never be without it – it has a big meaning for my identity – it is being a woman. Losing your sexuality is like losing a language, not only within your relationship but with other people. When you don't have a satisfactory sex life you lose an act of communication . . .'
Anna, aged 30, suffering from female sexual dysfunction.

Women – just like men – suffer from an inability to enjoy, desire or participate in sex with their partner. New research* in the UK and America suggests that as many as four in every ten women are affected by sexual dysfunction problems which is often described by them as 'female impotence'.

You may have wondered why you don't have that 'natural instinct' for sex other women describe. Or why you've lost the sexual spark you used to enjoy in your partner's presence? You may have even questioned your own sexual identity because you find it difficult, or even impossible, to become sexually aroused.

You may have gone through sexual therapy or counselling and perhaps even tried HRT. Doctors, possibly even partners, might have told you that what you are experiencing, however distressing, is 'all part of the ageing process', a 'natural consequence' of having a baby or changing your lifestyle, or simply that 'this is normal for you' –

***Note:** Some of the personal stories contained within this book are the testaments of women aged between 18 and 65 from the UK, America, Australia, Italy, France and Denmark, who at the time of interview were experiencing sexual problems, or had suffered them in the previous six months. Names have been changed to protect their anonymity. Their experiences were researched by Dr Frances Quirk, a health psychologist and sexual health advisor for Pfizer, the pharmaceutical company , who has used facts gleaned from their interviews to form the basis of the world's first study on how sexual problems fundamentally affect and influence the quality of women's sex lives today.*

opinion rather than diagnosis, which does nothing to solve the problem.

If you are suffering from female impotence you may never have had an orgasm, or felt sexually excited. You may once have enjoyed sex but now suffer unexplained pain on intercourse, a distressing lack of lubrication, even a complete loss of genital sensation. Despite these discomforts you may succumb to sex for the emotional 'reward' of the closeness or companionship of a partner but you may be beginning to dread the act.

You may struggle with what you think is a unique flaw in your sexuality which strikes at the heart of your relationships. But you cope by locking it away in the back of your mind ('nothing can be done so I'll put my energies into something else, like the children, or career').

Your partner may have been expressing some dissatisfaction too – because you never feel like initiating sex. (Unlike 30 years ago when men expected partners to be passive sexually, they now expect women to initiate too, and can complain when this does not happen)

This book reveals for the first time the deep well of unhappiness that exists among women whose sexual problems have not, until now, been fully recognised. Dr Quirk (*see note on facing page*) has tapped directly into this seam of despair. She has made a two-year study of the impact of sexual problems on the sex lives of women which has involved conducting personal interviews with 82 women in six countries followed by a random survey among a further 1,160 women in the UK.

Through these interviews she discovered the very real misery sexual problems cause women and the impact on not only them, but their relationships around them, their partners and their lifestyles. She has used this new material to report for the first time on the impact of sexual difficulties on the quality of life of modern women – focusing particularly on the social, physical, emotional and psychological consequences of sexual problems. Details of these findings are to be found later in this book. Her work, and new research by clinical specialists in sexual medicine both in the UK and

America, will provide the foundation for a radical new clinical approach to female sexual problems. It will undoubtedly mean that in the very near future the diagnostic 'bibles' used by clinicians will have to be changed to take into account new information about women's sexual response, sexuality and sexual difficulties.

Women of today who are part of the Pill generation and who are experiencing these problems in very great numbers, are demanding answers as to why their sex life has deteriorated. They believe that men have been sorted out with Viagra. It is now the turn of women to ask 'what about us?'.

And there is good reason. Sex education and therapy, combined with modern medication, is about to become increasingly available to women. It is now believed that a high proportion of female sexual problems may have a physical, biological cause – and medical science is breaking new ground in the quest for a complete understanding. For example, a woman who is unable to have an orgasm or has difficulty in feeling 'sexy' may have a condition recently identified as 'clitoral insufficiency' due to a poor or interrupted flow of blood to the erectile tissue of the clitoris. Or she may have a hormonal abnormality which puts the brakes on sexual drive.

An inability to lubricate might be triggered by specific impairments of the arterial circulation into the vagina which interferes with the normal vascular processes required for lovemaking.

There are other causes of female impotence, just as there are for erectile dysfunction in men – and these are linked with diabetes, multiple sclerosis (MS), high cholesterol levels, a narrowing of the arteries and heart disease, certain prescription drugs (particularly some anti-depressants), blood vessel or nerve damage from pelvic or abdominal surgery, such as hysterectomies, some gynaecological cancer treatments, even childbirth.

The very latest research indicates clearly that the biggest problems for women are 'loss of desire' and 'an inability, or difficulty, in becoming sexually aroused' although there are other symptoms such as pain on intercourse, a lack of lubrication and an inability to attain orgasm. These problems may be interlinked and may have several causes – possibly triggered by hormone imbalances or an underlying inefficiency of vital chemical messengers which all play a part in the female sexual response.

Some desire problems may be interconnected with psychological 'blocks': if there is pain on intercourse due to an underlying physiological problem then a 'lovesick' woman is likely to draw back from that pain next time and so a vicious cycle is created. You may need help not only to remove the physical 'stumbling block' but also help to overcome the 'pain barrier'.

Physiological female sexual arousal difficulties – 'female impotence' – have a direct parallel with erectile dysfunction in men because both conditions are caused by blood flow problems. The ground is now being prepared to acknowledge more fully and accept these sexual difficulties as medical conditions in their own right with their own answers and treatments.

The race is on among leading pharmaceutical companies, such as Pfizer and Harvard Scientific, to provide the first drug to help women regain their sexual feelings, restoring their lost desire and passion for an enjoyable love life.

Despite physiological similarities, there is a fundamental difference to male 'impotence' or erectile dysfunction, which makes the female equivalent of 'sexual arousal' problems – as well as the other sexual difficulties – more complex to manage medically.

On the whole, a woman's *emotional needs* also have to be met for good sex to occur – there has to be a psychological bonding. Women often engage in sex just to be close to their partners while men often seek sex for the absolute pleasure they derive from the mechanical act. Sex for a woman generally tends to be more of an expression of the relationship – and if a man cannot stimulate a woman in the right way, nor respond nor even understand her highly individual needs, she may suffer sexually.

New research indicates that an older woman may need to re-evaluate her sex life with her partner: after years together they may need to work on different ways to stimulate each other in order to avoid sex becoming a chore and dwindling to a halt.

One woman in her 50s said of her sexual difficulty: 'I've never really considered myself as getting old and now I can see different things happening to my body. The sex is not as often as it used to be so when we do have sex, I use a lubricant. After the lubrication and penetration then comes the dryness. It's not a comfortable feeling. At first I felt very down, I felt like something was missing, maybe I felt like I wasn't complete. The first time it happened I could not stand the penetration and I asked him to stop and I could see the hurt in his face.'

High-profile research and revelations during the last few years into male impotence has prompted the latest investigations into sexual dysfunction in women. But in the last 18 months the floodgates to new information – and a readiness to talk more freely about sexual problems – have opened. In the past year the Impotence Association has quite suddenly and dramatically begun to receive many calls from women asking for information about their sexual problems.

I predict that in the next few years we shall find more GPs and more specialists available to help women – and an eradication of the embarrassment which has prevented these conversations and consultations from taking place in the past. There will be more treatments available, from sex therapy for women, to drugs to treat specific physiological problems preventing women from enjoying a fulfilling sex life.

What we are currently witnessing is a cultural and social change: sexual problems are at last coming out of the closet, into the open. The question ' how many times a week is normal?' is being replaced with ' why aren't I having any joyful sex?' followed by 'what can be done to help?'

Some specialists in sexual medicine who have been working on resolving male impotence for the past 10 to 15 years now see their work more or less complete with the launch of medications like Viagra. Some of these same urologists and clinicians (and they do tend to be 'male' specialists rather than gynaecologists) are turning their attention to women. Until now sexual dysfunctions in women have received little notice – and most vitally, little funding. Female sexuality has been a male-dominated field with male views deciding what women want and desire. There is still some resistance to financing research at university level as it has been considered less important than other areas of health or quality of life studies.

Further, women's sexual problems have largely been ignored because it is a far more difficult problem to investigate. Research indicates that while men want a 'quick fix' for their problems, women want to increase their sexual desire or their libido in order to improve their relationships and this involves a more complex combination of mechanical and psychological factors.

But as sexual medicine advances (with the strong backing of pharmaceutical companies which recognise the potentially massive marketplace) new, improved ways have been found to measure female sexual response and so new discoveries are being made about women and for women. This is coupled with a demand for more information from women themselves – and the acknowledgment that these problems really do exist and they do affect quality of life.

Professor Edward Laumann says in a major report on sexual dysfunction published in 1999 in the *Journal of the American Medical Association*: 'The results . . . indicate that sexual problems are widespread in society and are influenced by both health-related and psychosocial factors. The role of the latter implies that stress inducing events due to either individual or social sources, can affect sexual functioning in both men and women . . . With the strong association between sexual dysfunction and impaired quality of life, this problem warrants recognition as a significant public health concern.'

This new line of work is in its early stages but it does show already that some arousal and sex drive problems encountered by large numbers of women have fundamental physical causes.

Viagra is already being prescribed to women in trials in Europe. The results of the first large series of clinical trials involving 700 women should be available by the end of 1999.

While this is at the cutting edge of medical research, there are other answers to sexual problems. This book examines some of them:

● the importance of understanding how and where women can be sexually stimulated: more information has come to light about erogenous zones
● the importance of exercise in stimulating sexual response.
● how low sexual desire might be helped with something as simple as watching a thrilling movie or drinking a cup of strong coffee – anything to stimulate the sympathetic nervous system
● how different lovemaking techniques and breathing exercises may help
● how testosterone may be the answer to many women's sexual problems. I report on success in the UK and Australia with testosterone implants.
● the influence of oestrogen rich foods, a change in diet, and use of herbs and aphrodisiacs.

Extraordinary as it may sound, one of the spin-offs from this fresh approach to female sexual dysfunction is a greater understanding of female physiology. Another is a deeper awareness of the complexities of female sexual arousal and female sexuality.

Some of it is so far reaching that anatomy text books may have to be re-written. This is explored in a special section of this book which explains, for the first time, the known elements of female sexual arousal, the latest discoveries concerning the clitoris and the role of the urethra, which is surrounded by 'erectile tissue' and effectively becomes a sexual organ in women.

why now?

Research into women's sexual problems is about 10 years behind the research into male impotence. There is a growing demand for help and information from women themselves who are now ready to speak up about their problems which range from never having experienced an orgasm to a complete loss of desire, or drive, to avoiding sex with their partner even though that partner may be deeply loved.

Sex today is seen as an important part of a woman's overall health and well-being.* There is no doubt that a good sex life enhances quality of life and, according to Dr Beverly Whipple who rediscovered the G-spot, sex also 'fosters personal growth and contributes to human fulfillment'.

She writes: 'When the term sexuality is viewed holistically it refers to the totality of being. It refers to human qualities and not just to the genitals and their functions. It includes all the qualities – biological, psychological, emotional, cultural, social and spiritual – that makes people who they are.'

In essence women today should expect to have a good sex life and be able to receive help if they are not having one. This is a fundamentally new and different approach to this most private and intimate part of our lives. In the past women have tended to complain about the more 'subjective' qualities of the sexual experience rather than specific physiological difficulties, says Dr John Bancroft, head of the Kinsey Institute in the US. The most common complaints have been loss of sexual desire, loss of enjoyment of sex, difficulty in reaching orgasm, and pain during intercourse.

The problem until recently was how to evaluate sexual arousal in a woman in laboratory conditions. New technology has produced the answers and there is now a range of instruments which can be used to measure blood movement and blood volume in the vagina, indicating levels of physiological arousal in a woman – just as an erect penis indicates arousal in a man.

In addition new questionnaires are currently being devised which will help to identify whether women are suffering from a sexual dysfunction problem – and if they are, what to do about it.

This form of 'self-evaluation' was used to determine how successful Viagra might be for men with erectile dysfunction problems, and has become a recognised way of evaluating certain conditions – especially sexual problems which can be influenced by artificial laboratory or clinical conditions or invasive laboratory techniques.

Women, deluged with information about progress on male impotence are coming forward to say they too have a fundamental problem which affects their health and lifestyle. Rather than put up with it as their mother's generation might have preferred to do, possibly encouraged by their embarrassed husbands or medical advisers, today's women are asking in no uncertain terms what their doctors are going to do about it.
Beyond the G Spot by Beverly Whipple and Prof. Barry Komisaruk, *Medical Aspects of Human Sexuality*, June 1998.

● ●

Accepting that some women's sexual problems are physical disorders which can be treated will have enormous repercussions. Doctors will have to be prepared for the floodgates to open as women ask for help and new drugs come onto the market for the first time. New assessment methods will have to be formulated and in some areas this is already starting to happen.

Female sexual dysfunction is thought to be a far more common problem than erectile dysfunction in men, affecting as many as four or five in 10 women (compared to one in 10 men for erectile dysfunction). This book sets out to explain what sexual dysfunction really means – and what treatments are already available.

summary
Specialists working in the high profile world of sexual medicine agree that female impotence tends to be more complex than male impotence and contrary to popular opinion affects younger women more than older women.

This book explains the key causes and examines the cures; including ways women can help themselves 'heal' their sexual dysfunction and go on to have happy and vastly improved sex lives.

This book should help thousands of women across the UK by revealing for the first time that they are not alone with their problems, that what they are feeling is not abnormal and that there are very many other women who are similarly affected.

further reading and information
Sexual Dysfunction in the United States by Prof. Edward Laumann and Dr Raymond Rosen, Professor of Psychiatry, Robert Wood Johnson Medical School, *Journal of the American Medical Association*.

Kinsey Institute – Information Services
Morrison Hall 302
Bloomington, IN 47405, USA
Tel 812/855-3037. Fax 812/855-8277

acknowledgments
Dr Roy Levin, Dr Frances Quirk, Prof. Alan Riley, Victoria Lehman, Margaret Ramage, Ann Craig, Relate, the Impotence Association, Dr Ellen Laan and Malcolm Whitehead.

CHAPTER ONE
....
what is female impotence?

'I feel I have lost my femininity and womanhood. I can't have sex and I am unable to have children and – and it's left me feeling empty,' – Susan, aged 54.

Traditionally, women have remained quiet about their sexual problems, putting up with them without too much complaint. Consequently, until fairly recently, women with sexual problems were simply not taken seriously or frequently labelled 'frigid' . Even so, there is little public awareness that women can experience sexual dysfunction as a direct result of disease, or arterial, neurological or hormonal problems. Part of the reason is that female sexual dysfunction has not been considered by the medical profession as a serious enough disorder to warrant much time or energy – until now, when the implications for possible new treatments are so clearly on the horizon.

Despite pioneering work by famous sexologists Kinsey and Masters and Johnson in the 1960s, the full story of what happens during female sexual arousal is still not completely understood. Accurate information about what happens is still badly lacking, although continuing research is breaking new ground.
There is even some confusion about basic physiology.
In 1998, Helen O'Connell, an Australian urologist, suggested that anatomy textbooks should be re-written following her discoveries about the size, positioning and functioning of the clitoris and its connection to the erectile tissue surrounding the urethra.
Advances in understanding are happening now because of more thorough investigation into physiological changes that occur before, during and after arousal and the use of scientific instruments to monitor these changes.

'We had a very active sex life at the beginning and now I feel frustrated, cheated, I have decreased self-worth, I feel asexual, less feminine, and afraid that my partner will leave me. Will I be able to give him the feeling that I love him in an unrestricted and uninhibited way . . .' – Julie, aged 40.

With no obvious erection stating 'yes, I am aroused' or 'no, I am not', women's sexual feelings have been considered far more subjective or controlled by their emotions. The direct parallel to erectile dysfunction, which affects one in 10 men is 'female arousal difficulty', the most common sexual problem for women. As you cannot see the complication as clearly as with erectile dysfunction, doctors might have told women in the past their sexual problems were 'all in the head'.

The added problem is that unlike men with erectile dysfunction, women can still 'function' sexually and have intercourse even if they feel disinterested.

Women experience swelling of erectile tissue during sexual arousal – they are not exactly erections as the tissues do not become rigid like an erect penis, but they certainly enlarge as the blood flows in. This flow of blood into the genitals provides medical researchers with an opportunity to learn about the female sexual response. There are now instruments which monitor the blood velocity and movement which create this tumescence.

The direct equivalent to a penis erecting is a woman lubricating and vaginal tissues swelling as blood pumps into these erectile tissues which surround the urethra, clitoris, vagina and labial folds. It is thought that the same chemicals responsible for a man's erection might control this response which is why treatments like Viagra or Vasofem might, in the future, be a solution for some women who have certain sexual arousal problems (although at this stage it is unlikely to be as great a solution as it is for men with erectile dysfunction problems).

For example, it may be possible to help women with special problems like arterial disease or diabetes where an improved blood flow to the vagina and genitals may help the sexual response.

However, clinical trials may find that for Viagra to work, a woman will have to be able to become aroused: it won't be a question of popping a pill and waiting for the magic to happen. The irony is that lack of sexual arousal and loss of sexual interest are the number one problems affecting women. How clinicians will get over this hurdle remains to be seen, but, as this book explains in later chapters, more avenues of treatment are opening up and women may be able to learn 'self-help' techniques to improve their sexual arousability.

sexual arousal

Researchers at the University of Amsterdam describe the female sexual response as a 'complicated bio-psychosocial' phenomenon.

Psychologist Dr Ellen Laan says she believes arousal is triggered by a combination of external and internal stimulation (touch, smell, the sight of a loved one or sexual thoughts and fantasy) influenced by the central and the peripheral nervous system. This induces a need to participate in sex to satisfy the 'drive.'

New research in the States suggests the vagus nerve which winds down through the body may be a 'sexual super highway' of the nervous system.

The result of this double, inter-connected stimulation is a cascade of biochemical, hormonal and circulatory changes in the body which lead to the feeling associated with sexual arousal – the tingling, warmth, and nipple erection.

Sex hormones, or more specifically certain component parts, play a vital part in arousal and excitement. They act on sensory organs and can determine libido – the motivational force for sex. The clitoris, labia and even nipples are constructed of androgen-dependent tissues and, although testosterone is generally considered to be a male hormone it is produced by the ovaries in women and is the 'fuel' which triggers the sex drive through its stimulating action upon androgen dependent tissues

As we age, levels of testosterone drop, and a shortage or imbalance may explain why some women do not experience sexual feelings (see chapter five – the testosterone story).

The next phase in this high speed chain reaction is a flow of blood to the genitals triggered by chemical messengers and the nervous system which responds within 20 seconds of an erotic thought. This leads to engorgement of the vagina – which triggers lubrication via the blood vessels – and the swelling of the clitoris and tissue around the urethra – the equivalent of a penis erecting.

Binding all these changes and influences are a woman's emotions, feelings or thoughts which can act as an override switch, turning off all the physical reactions as quickly as they were turned on. Previous sexual experiences can also play a part: some women need help to remove links between sexual response and negative feelings of guilt, anger or disgust.

how big is the problem?

'I find that not being able to have sex is a terrible loss – being interviewed about sex makes me recall how good things used to be – it's strange because my life is happy in all other areas and I'm happier than I've ever been. I feel that a part of my life has vanished.' – Anita, aged 53, suffering from female sexual dysfunction.

'We are of the generation where wives are expected to please their husbands and if I don't want sex with him then he thinks it must be because I am wanting sex with someone else. I have tried to explain to my husband and he is getting better but I think we'll both be dead before he understands . . .'. – Maria, aged 33, suffering from a loss of interest in sex.

'My sexual feelings have closed off. I have become more shy. I have guilt feelings and a loss of self-worth and identity – I don't feel like a woman.' – Celine, in her 30s, who has 'lost' her sexual feeling.

Sex is a vitally important part of a fulfilling and loving relationship, often considered to be the cement, or the bonding. When sex goes wrong for a woman it can damage the very core of her closest relationship and the very heart of her self-esteem. The American study involved candid interviews with 1,749 women and 1,410 men aged between 18 and 59. The startling conclusion was that younger women are more likely to have problems with sexual desire and arousal than older women (apart from those who have trouble with lubrication leading to the problems of a dry vagina).

A total of 43% of women reported significant problems with sexual desire, arousal or orgasm compared to 31% of men. Happiness, it suggested, is a key factor in a happy sex life. Emotional and physical satisfaction with the partner were of prime importance along with 'feelings of general happiness'.

young and old

Unmarried women are 1.5 times as likely to have sexual problems involving orgasm and sexual anxiety than married women. A US report suggests that women in stable relationships and long-term marriages enjoy their sex lives better than young women who may have a high incidence of 'partner turnover.'

The extent of the problem means there are potentially very many unhappy and sexually unfulfilled young and single women, most of whom are not aware they may be helped. It has been estimated that there are around 50 women of all ages in every GP's practice in the country who might need help for a sexual problem.

Prof. Alan Riley, the UK's first professor of sexual medicine at the University of Central Lancashire in Preston, conducted a pilot study among 100 women and found that 30% of women reported they had no sex drive whatsoever.

He also discovered there are two peak ages for problems: the 30s and the 50s, confirming the US finding. Another survey by genito-urinary specialists at St. Mary's Hospital in London revealed that 60% of the women interviewed had experienced some sort of sexual problem – 22% reported problems with orgasm and 25% with vaginismus (a spasm of the vaginal muscles which blocks the entrance to the vagina). Around two-thirds said they would like to have treatment, one-third said they would not.

The first full population survey* of the extent and nature of sexual problems in the UK has shown how common they are – affecting 41% of women – that is four women in every 10. Only a small number had had help for their problem – although a large number wanted help. The survey was carried out in four GP practices in England among 789 men and 979 women and concluded:

- one-third of the respondents had not had sex in the previous three months
- 41% of women reported having one or more sexual problems during the previous three months
- the most common female problems were: vaginal dryness and orgasm difficulties
- sexual intercourse was never or rarely a pleasant experience for 110 of the women
- 68% reported having some sort of sexual problem at some time previously
- but only 4% of women had received help

The problem is widespread: yet very little is being done for affected women – partly because so few seek help as women are not sure where to go. Apart from the GP, or the genito-urinary clinic, or sexual and marital therapists who take a largely 'psychological' approach, there are very few clinics offering specific sexual help for women from a medical perspective. Little attention is paid to the fact that women may also feel happier talking to another woman about these problems.

what is sexual dysfunction for a woman?

Two years of research by Dr Quirk has tapped into a 'great well of unhappiness' being endured by women with sex problems; many of whom feel their condition is not being adequately dealt with or even properly understood by either their partners or their doctors.

*Source: Association of sexual problems with social, psychological and physical problems in men ad women: a cross-sectional survey, *Journal of Epidemiology and Community Health*, March 1999, Vol.53 No.3, pp144-148

She has conducted the world's first study into the impact of sex problems on women's sexual quality of life. Her ground-breaking findings will lead to a greater understanding of women's sexual dysfunction – and, along with work being conducted in the US and elsewhere, may contribute to a new clinical description of the disorder for doctors. Her research involved interviews and surveys with 1,242 women and discloses for the first time the extent of the suffering endured by women with sexual problems and the impact on their sex lives and relationships.

She conducted or supervised 82 face-to-face detailed and often highly emotional interviews with women. Some women had kept their problems and feelings bottled up for a long time and wept openly about the poor state of their sex lives, which was directly affecting them and their close relationships, as well as feelings of insecurity about their partners. Many women felt disempowered, and were deeply hurt that their self-worth and self-esteem were irreparably damaged. Others were worried that their husbands would leave them.

From these interviews, Dr Quirk developed a questionnaire which was randomly sent out to 1,160 women. More than 72% replied and of those, an astounding 400 said they had recently suffered or were suffering one of six sexual problems listed in the questionnaire.

Dr Quirk was particularly keen to find out about difficulties with sexual arousal and loss of sexual interest in a partner – because these are described by women as the major problems in almost every survey sexual health survey in the UK or USA.

Her work confirmed this:
● 50% of women who said they had sexual problems said they suffered or had suffered a recent 'lack of interest' in sex
● 30% said they took a long time to become aroused and another 26% said they had difficulty becoming aroused

Other complaints were:
● lack of lubrication (24%)
● pain or discomfort having sex (35%)
● difficulty achieving orgasm (28%)

The sexual quality of life survey focused on the impact of the social, physical, emotional and psychological consequences of sexual problems and concluded that large numbers of women simply do not have satisfactory sex lives. Many women who have arousal or loss of interest problems have a very poor quality of life sexually.

The survey reveals that
● a quarter of women with sexual arousal problems do not find their sexual life an enjoyable part of their life overall
● nearly 30% are not satisfied with the frequency of sex
● nearly 1 in 5 of the women had lost all pleasure in sex
● a third of the women worried about the future of their sex lives

As this was a random survey the women who returned their questionnaires were ordinary women in the UK – a cross-section – and, because of this, these results undoubtedly reflect what is happening in the lives of any given group of 1,000 women in the UK. Of the women who responded 80% had a partner, 96% had had a relationship in the past six months and 84% had children.

In other words the sex lives of many women in this country seem to be in a shocking state – yet there are few clinics or clinicians available to help. Indeed many women do not think they can be helped. Not surprisingly, the survey also revealed that over 40% of women with sexual problems avoid having sex and worry about their future sex lives.

An interesting insight into women's understanding of sexual problems was shown by the 5 to 10% of women who said they have never had a sexual problem but who added that they do not consider sex to be an enjoyable part of their life, overall.

how the research was conducted
In order to find out about how sex problems influence women's sexual quality of life, Dr Quirk devised a questionnaire that could be understood by them, using words they would use to describe their sexual problems.

She initially interviewed 82 women in six different countries – 22 of whom had sought help for sexual problems although the interviews also disclosed that a further 12 had one or more of the key sexual problems – such as a loss of arousal, lack of interest, problems with attaining orgasm, lubrication difficulty or pain on intercourse although they had not sought help.

It was through these one to one interviews that she tapped deep into the heart of the problem and faced, for the first time, the enormity of the problem and the unhappiness a life without sex can mean. It has an impact on the women, and their families: possibly even the family structure. Many women worried their husbands would leave them because of their problem – a lack of interest in sex, or an inability to feel sexually aroused.

Why women complain in such large numbers about their loss of interest in partners, or 'going off sex' is at the heart of all the current work and research on sexual dysfunction in women. But at the time of writing it still remains something of a medical mystery – although more answers to this will come as scientists and clinicians focus on the problem.

What is new is the wider recognition and acceptance of the fact that a large proportion of women suffer from sexual dysfunction at some stage in their lives. This recognition is only just starting to filter down to doctors, and, most importantly affected women themselves.

The next step will be finding solutions to it – and whether that will be in the form of a pink diamond-shaped pill to complement the blue diamond-shape of Viagra for men remains to be seen.

Dr Quirk began her quest by finding out what women thought about sexual arousal and arousal problems. 'I wanted to know what they deemed sexual arousal to be and what were women's signals for becoming sexually aroused? I wanted to know about 'the normal sexual response' in women and what women consider sexual arousal to mean, before moving on to find out about the impact of female sexual dysfunction on women's sexual quality of life. I was interested in how women described these signals and what language they used.'

Giving new insight into the problem, she concludes: 'Sexual arousal for a man is not necessarily the same as sexual arousal for a woman. There are many interlinking factors for women. For women, sexual arousal may be far more complex and both sexual interest and arousal are more deeply interrelated than has been previously understood.

'One of the things which became clear is that the signals women use are both emotional and psychological. They might mention that arousal means being more lubricated, they are more sensitive to touch but they also mention that they felt much closer to their partner and the emotional side which was just as important as the physical side in terms of feeling aroused, before they embarked on sex.'

What the result of the research will mean
Dr Quirk's work is part of a move towards a greater understanding of female sexual response and female sexual dysfunction. It may lead to new clinical definitions and possible future treatments.

Terms and definitions
Female sexual dysfunctions are currently classified as discrete disorders in one of the phases of the sexual response cycles – desire, arousal, orgasm, resolution/satisfaction – or pain related to sexual activity. The problems have led to the current terms 'drive disorder', 'female sexual arousal disorder', 'female orgasm disorder' and 'pain disorder'.

These are the terms and descriptions used in the Diagnostics and Statistical Manual (DSM1V), a psychiatric diagnostic manual used by clinicians.

But Dr Quirk's work talking to real women with real problems reveals how much more interrelated the phases are than previously recognised. She believes that one difficulty is that female sexual dysfunction disorders are separated too much into distinct classifications.

'We need to come up with different definitions for female sexual dysfunctions because these are not necessarily discrete disorders where the effect is on only one phase of the sexual response cycle.

'A woman who says I am not interested in sex any more could be someone who has a fundamental drive disorder or an inter-connected arousal disorder or a secondary complication of a condition they have already.

'Desire and arousal for example are not separate phases, they are interrelated and each one feeds back on the other. There is a loop rather than a move from one distinct phase to the next. For example, a disorder in the arousal phase will have an effect on a woman's level of interest or willingness to engage in sex with a partner.'

Her work has also highlighted the lack of information and knowledge that is available to women. During interviews, she found most women put sexual problems down to such factors as 'going off my partner', 'having a baby' or 'getting older'. Few thought that sexual dysfunction might be caused by an illness or a physical problem.

'There was a great lack of knowledge especially among women who had never experienced a sexual difficulty.'

men versus women : their different perspectives on sexual desire

The new research has confirmed what women have anecdotally believed for years: that women do have quite different needs – and ideas – about sex than men. If these needs are not addressed, problems result which can impact upon their lives as a whole.

- Men's sexual desire is largely governed by a strong biological drive, reinforced with the external signs of an erection.
- Women's sexual desire has a stronger psychological and emotional input which can be just as important as physical feelings, and possibly better recognised than the physiological changes of blood flow and vaginal ballooning associated with sexual arousal.
  A woman, says Dr Quirk, will be much more interested in the person with whom she is involved sexually and will respond to 'focused desire' which means she will usually have to be interested in being close to that person. Women tend to be more aware of these thoughts about

a partner than they are of the physical changes taking place.

Any future measurement of female sexual dysfunction will inevitably have to take into account the thoughts and emotions a woman experiences when she is having problems with sex.

Dr Quirk discovered that the problems women faced with their sexuality knew no national boundaries – there were no cultural differences separating the women. Those who felt living without joyful sex was a deep loss, she says, were all desperately seeking a solution to what, until now, has been their 'secret' and hidden problem, largely misunderstood not only by doctors but also their partners.

It is easy to diagnose erectile dysfunction in a man but how do women recognise the symptoms of female arousal disorders?
When it comes to sex do you:
- **have internal physical reactions such as warmth, tingling and genital sensations?**
- **experience sexual fantasies, thoughts and images?**
- **have interest in your sexual partner?**
- **interest in non-genital touch or behaviour?**
If the answer is 'no' to all these questions, then you may be experiencing an arousal disorder.

Formulating a questionnaire defining sexual dysfunction will not only help researchers to understand the extent of the problem – and how women view it – but also will be used in determining how successful new therapies might be.

Female sexual dysfunction (FSD) is a global expression covering a wide range of sexual problems affecting women. FSD is not straightforward as Dr Quirk's research proves. But there are various disorders which are usually explored by clinicians although an affected woman may suffer from one or a combination of these conditions. Few sexologists like the term 'impotence' because it is seen as a negative phrase and technically a definition of male erectile dysfunction. However, women do often use this word to describe their symptoms, according to the Impotence Association.

1) lack of sexual drive

It is estimated that 30% of women with sexual dysfunction problems have no sex drive – the biological force which makes someone seek out or accept sex. Affected women have no need for sex (unless, notably, they want to have a baby). A zero sex drive is most likely to have a biological, or physical, explanation. This is a new finding and it is pushing forward the research into treatments and causes.

Note: *women with no sex drive have no interest in participating in sex – although they often will have sex to achieve a closeness with their man, or to seek touch of a partner without the penetration.*

symptoms
● no desire to initiate sex
● no desire to participate in sex unless trying for a baby but may seek comfort from cuddling alone without penetration
● pain on intercourse due to a dry vagina
● lack of feeling or stimulation in the clitoris
● inability to become properly stimulated or reach orgasm

possible physical causes
● neurological impairment, possibly after pelvic or gynaecological surgery
● insufficient blood flow to the clitoris or vagina
● low testosterone levels
● high blood pressure
● thyroid disease
● high prolactin levels (the hormone which circulates during breast feeding)
● alcohol or drug problems
● diabetes

tests
● hormone levels checked
● thyroid function monitored
● biofeedback to monitor blood flow

treatments
- use of hormonal creams
- treatment for an underlying condition, such as thyroid problems or diabetes
- oxytocin – researchers are looking at whether it may be a useful pro-sexual drug in women

2) lack of sexual desire or ISD (inhibited sexual desire)

The number of women with reduced sexual desire has increased 'substantially' over the past 20 years, according to Prof. Alan Riley, chairman of the Impotence Association. It is the most frequent complaint among women attending sex therapy clinics affecting 80% of women who seek help.

Women who lose their desire may not have lost their drive and may be quite capable of having good sex with orgasm. They may 'learn' to lose interest in sex because of pain, a bad experience or something off-putting – it could as simple as a partner having dirty fingernails. Women who lose their sexual desire may still want to be held by their partners and 'loved' but may not want penetration. However, this signal can be wrongly misinterpreted by the partner as a desire for sex leading to a build up of hostility and then guilt. Loss of sexual desire can be confused with loss of drive: tests can show a woman that she is responding in the right way physically and help her to recognise those feelings.

symptoms
- loss of sexual spark
- little desire to initiate sex although if stimulated properly can still achieve orgasm
- aversion to sexual overtures
- dyspareunia – or pain on intercourse
- distress or emotional upset
- inability to respond to stimulation or maintain lubrication

possible causes
- extreme tiredness
- depression or use of certain anti-depressants
- androgen deficiency (after hysterectomy, removal of ovaries, or

chemotherapy for cancer)
- alcohol or drug abuse
- urological, obstetric or gynaecological complications which cause pain when having sex such as vaginismus and vestibulitis
- a psychological block because of a previous bad experience or parental influence
- obesity and loss of self-esteem
- general unhappiness in relationships or with partner
- stress or anxiety with work or home
- unresolved sexual orientation
- previous traumatic sexual experience
- the contraceptive pill can sometimes inhibit desire

tests
- hormone levels checked
- assessment of anti-depressant drugs
- gynaecological check up
- review of contraception

treatments
- psycho-sexual counselling
- testosterone treatment
- a change in type and hormonal content of the birth pill
- alcohol or drugs counselling
- weight loss plan
- stimulation of the sympathetic nervous system – through exercise or 'excitement' which raises blood pressure and heart rate

3) lack of sexual arousal or FSAD (female sexual arousal disorder)

Female sexual arousal disorder can occur on its own, or in combination with either of the other two problems. It is very likely to have a physical cause and new research has defined two problems – vascular and clitoral erectile insufficiency syndrome: which means that arterial disease might influence blood flow and the subsequent required engorgement of clitoral, vaginal and urethral tissues.

Like men with erectile dysfunction, women's sexual responses can sometimes fail because of a physical problem in the complex sexual circuitry. During normal arousal a woman's clitoris, and the tissues surrounding the vaginal opening become engorged with blood rather like a penis does. The clitoris has the same nerve endings as a penis, and enlarges during arousal. At the same time the vagina elongates to receive the penis. Furthermore, physiologists now believe that in normal arousal the erectile tissues around the urethra expand to produce pleasurable sensations. It is perhaps not surprising: both male and female genitals develop from the same sort of fetal tissue (anlagen, a German word meaning 'the same) which in maturity reacts in a similar way to sexual stimulation.

symptoms
● an inability to lubricate – leading to vaginal dryness – affecting mostly older women
● no 'erotic sensations' or feelings of heightened sexual excitement
● no orgasm (anorgasmia)
● pain with intercourse
● diminished vaginal sensation

possible causes
● physiological complication such as an impairment of the blood flow to the clitoris or vagina or nerve damage around the urethra, vagina, or clitoris
● lack of adequate stimulation from partner/lack of ability to arouse partner
● arterial or vascular disease
● chronic disease such as epilepsy, kidney failure
● multiple sclerosis
● hormonal changes at the menopause
● pelvic injury damaging the arteries leading to the vagina and clitoris restricting the blood flow.

tests
● Doppler imaging to monitor blood changes in the genitalia
● blood tests for chronic illness
● hormonal checks
● nerve assessment

treatments
● combined HRT and methyl testosterone (still considered controversial by some doctors)

- change in diet
- vitamin, mineral or herbal supplements
- improved happiness through relaxation and exercise
- alternative therapies
- change in sexual techniques and new sexual stimulation
- topical vaginal oestrogens for peri- and post-menopausal women
- artificial lubricants, such as KY-jelly

the future

new drugs to improve sexual arousal – still in trials
Viagra (sildenafil) or Vasomax (phentolamine) may particularly help menopausal women – if they are approved (not expected before year 2001).

The first study of the effects of Viagra on women was published in the US journal, *Urology* in March 1999. Dr Steven Kaplan, a professor of urology at the Columbia University College of Physicians and Surgeons tested the drug on 33 post-menopausal women in stable relationships – each woman took a 50mg of the drug one hour before planned sexual activity. The most common problem reported by the women was of low sexual arousal.

The effectiveness of the Viagra therapy was analysed at four, eight and 12 weeks – and the results showed that there was no significant change either in 'intercourse satisfaction or in the degree of sexual desire' after the women had taken Viagra for 12 weeks. However, 25% of the patients had some improvement in overall sexual functioning and 21% had a 'significant response'. Clitoral sensation improved by 31% and lubrication by 23%. Interestingly, however, only 20 per cent of patients wanted to continue after 12 weeks. Dr Kaplan suggests that Viagra did appear to increase blood flow to the clitoris but this did not seem to translate to increased sexual satisfaction. 'Neither increased clitoral sensation or lubrication would be expected to be of benefit to women with diminished desire to either initiate or respond to sexual activity. Clearly, relationships are important and this needs to be further investigated,' he says.

Prostaglandin E cream; one study has shown that it can increase clitoral blood flow but more studies are required. A US company is on the brink of launching a prostaglandin pill as a treatment for female sexual dysfunction and, they claim, 'provide a solution to the problem of a dry vagina' by increasing blood flow to the genitals. Prostaglandin E-1 is already marketed for male erectile dysfunction as a vasodilator and administered by needle injection in Upjohn's Caverject product but Harvard Scientific Corporation believes that in women, it will increase vaginal lubrication for intercourse as well as encourage heightened sexual sensation.

Androgen therapy (testosterone) for post-menopausal women (**see chapter five, testosterone – the hormone of desire?**)

Apormorphine: this is a drug well known to medicine and used mainly in the past as an emetic, to induce vomiting. However, it can be combined with other drugs to prevent the nausea it triggers and research is currently underway to find out whether it has a role in the treatment of both male and female impotence. Apormorphine probably works by increasing the level of certain chemical messengers such as dopamine in the brain: Oliver Gillie in his book *Regaining Potency* (Self-Help Direct, 1997) says that in the future it will probably be used together with drugs like Viagra – with one drug working on the brain and the other on the blood flow to the penis (in men) or the clitoris in women.

There are currently 11 pharmaceutical companies interested in developing treatments for female sexual dysfunction. Testosterone implants are an approved treatment – but may only help a small proportion of affected women. Things are likely to change rapidly within the next five years and a number of breakthroughs are expected.

factors needed for good sex

physical
- genital response
- no pain
- engorgement through blood flow to the vagina, clitoris and labia
- correct levels of testosterone, the hormone which affects the sex drive

- healthy, working sensory nerves to provide and send the pleasurable feelings to the brain via spinal cord
- lubrication to aid penetration – otherwise it will be painful. The blood flow to the vagina facilitates lubrication.

psychological or emotional
- psychological empathy, 'desire' or emotional contact with partner
- the 'drive' or need to participate in sex with a partner
- the need to feel comfortable with what is happening, free of anxiety, anger and distraction.
- an ability to let go and enjoy the experience without 'sex guilt'

If these basics are not in place the outcome is:
- dry vagina and pain
- inadequate engorgement of the labia, making vaginal opening difficult
- if the uterus is not elevated during intercourse, the cervix tends to stay 'fixed in one place, and this coupled with poor vaginal engorgement will lead to painful buffeting of the cervix.
- reduced genital sensation
- no response to sexual stimulus
- no desire to want to make love
● ●

what women really, really want
Researchers at the Robert Wood Johnson Medical School in New Jersey, USA make the pertinent point that doctors should consider what women really want from 'sex'. For many women sexual satisfaction includes affection, communication with their partner, and sensual touching and they say that attraction, passion, trust and intimacy are more significant than their genital response. Some women find that specific problems can put them off sex, and cause them to lose their desire for sex.

these problems include:
Painful intercourse (dyspaurenia) can range from a sharp,

burning sensation to a very deep pain to an external burning sensation. The deep and burning pain is often because of a lack of lubrication, which is discussed in a later chapter, or other causes including endometriosis. There may be pain if there is failure of the womb to rise and the vagina to balloon to accommodate the penis, or when there is pelvic inflammatory disease or prolapsed ovaries. External vaginal pain may be caused by a condition called vestibulitis, an inflammatory problem, genital herpes, or an acute infection of the vagina. There may be sensitivity to contraceptive creams or devices such as the cap, even condoms. Diabetic women are prone to thrush which can cause soreness and irritation. Occasionally cysts can develop which in turn can become painful abscesses.

This sort of pain can lead to sexual dysfunction because the pain becomes a vicious circle – when sex equals pain there is a reluctance to try again. The pain needs to be resolved but the woman may then need extra help to overcome the association between pain and sex.

vaginismus
This problem involves the muscles of the pelvic floor which surrounds the vagina – if the muscles tense up it makes vaginal entry difficult. Some women experience an uncontrolled spasm which effectively cuts off entry to the vagina and may arch their back as if trying to escape. A woman who repeatedly suffers from this can inevitably be put off sex, even though their drive may still be intact. There may be a psychological association- which could be linked to a past trauma – such as rape or abuse – which triggers this response. There is often a link with painful intercourse. Anxiety, involuntary muscle contractions, problems with sexual excitement, lubrication and lack of desire can all contribute.

vestibulitis
More is being understood about this condition which is an inflammation causing considerable pain around the vagina.

lack of genital response
Some women complain that their clitoris feels 'dead' and they have no pleasurable feelings from touching the clitoris. These same women may also suffer dry vaginas.

female orgasmic disorder (FOD)

Some women complain of not being able to achieve orgasm even though they do feel sexually aroused and responsive. This is a common problem – second only to sexual arousal disorders. The problem for clinicians is establishing what is 'normal' – female orgasmic ability varies hugely. Some women can become orgasmic with nipple stimulation and fantasy; others need long periods of clitoral stimulation; and yet others are never able to achieve orgasm. There is probably a significant psychological element in orgasm disorders (**see chapter three: sex and the mind**).

further help:

The Impotence Association, Tel 0181-767-7791 weekdays between 9am and 5pm. Or write to the association at PO Box 10296, London SW12 9WH. At the time of writing a special section for women was being planned to provide information and advice to women with sexual dysfunctions needing help.

Vulval Pain Society, PO Box 514, Slough, Berkshire, SL1 2BP. Information and advice on all vulval diseases, including dietary treatments and explanations of the conditions.

CHAPTER TWO
....
sex and physiology

'If I met someone who said that I could regain my sexual feelings, I would do almost anything – I'd say, let's go for it. But as time goes by I've rationalized my feelings – this is where I am now,' – Martine, aged in her 60s, suffering from an inability to become sexually aroused.

Scientists are still pushing forward frontiers of understanding about female physiology in relation to sex and sexual responses. One woman researcher working in the field summed up the general lack of knowledge as 'woefully horrendous'.

Despite greater openness about sexuality today many women have very little understanding of their own bodies or exactly what happens during sexual arousal. This chapter aims to explain a little more about the interconnected physical responses and also how they are linked to our emotions and psychological responses.

To understand the disorders of female impotence and sexual dysfunction it helps to understand what happens during the normal response. Although research is still on going and parts of the jigsaw puzzle are falling into place, Helen O'Connell, based at the Royal Melbourne Hospital in Australia, says that 'more systematic physiological studies are required'.

Drug companies currently employ some of the most eminent doctors and scientists working in sexual medicine to test the effectiveness of Viagra for women and to find out more about the physiology of females: it has taken these powerful drug companies to realise that there is a huge untapped market of women who might benefit from drugs to alleviate their sexual dysfunction.

Taking a different view are psychologists trying to determine the importance of the mind and the brain in the arousal process and a woman's ability to 'let go' or lose control during sex which they believe is equally as important as the mechanical aspects. This is explored more in **chapter three: sex and the mind**.

Even 10 years ago, erectile dysfunction in men was thought to be mainly psychological except in the obvious cases of paralysis and injury. But now it is acknowledged that between 70 and 90 per cent of cases have a physical cause. This discovery has launched a new industry: Viagra and Viagra-like products – which, it is estimated, can help 70% of affected men.
But will it do the same for women?
A few women with certain problems connected with blood flow to and engorgement of the genitals may be helped, particularly if the drugs are given in conjunction with psychotherapy. But unless you are one of the women involved in trials currently underway it is unlikely that any drugs for female impotence will become available much before the year 2001. Even then it is unlikely they will be able to provide 'instant orgasms' – sildenfil, otherwise known as Viagra, requires sexual stimulation, or arousal, before it works.
There are already clinicians in America who are convinced that it does help women and say they have already had success prescribing it unofficially for women.
Making new drugs for women has a number of extra-ethical questions – for example, could they harm a woman during pregnancy?

In the beginning ...

In the womb we are all alike for the first six to eight weeks. One genital tubercle exists which will form the penis in a boy or the clitoris in a girl.
The Y chromosome is the switch which creates the testes from this 'indifferent gonad', an 'ovotestis' which can develop into either male or female sexual organs. In boys the fetal testis then secretes testosterone which acts locally to support and differentiate the Wolffian ducts

which make the male 'plumbing', and via the blood, to the
external genital tubercle which develops into the penis.
The fetal testis also makes a chemical which inhibits the
development of the so-called Mullerian duct which
develops into the female genitals.
In boys, the genital tubercle grows into the penis which
grows outwards. The scrotal and urethral folds fuse
together to form the scrotum
In girls, the genital tubercle becomes the clitoris which, it
is now known, grows inwards and is also inter-connected
to the urethra. The tissue which becomes the scrotum in
boys becomes the inner and outer labial folds.
In maturity there are two types of erectile tissue which
engorge upon sexual stimulation.
The *corpus cavernosa* is the tissue which provides the
erection in men and the swelling of the clitoris in women.
The *corpus spongiosum* surrounds the urethra in men and
is 'sponge-like' and in women this type of tissue surrounds
the vaginal bulbs and glans of the clitoris.

● ●

the key elements of sexual arousal

Dr Roy Levin is a physiologist at Sheffield University and has been
studying the female sexual response for almost 30 years. His work is
considered to be some of the most detailed of its kind and a
reference point for much of the new wave of research.

Dr Levin suggests that some women may suffer sexually because they
are simply not being stimulated effectively by their partners due to:
● a lack of awareness (by both partners) of the female genital
  anatomy
● what happens during arousal
● and where the important sexually arousable zones are
  positioned

Although there is awareness of the G-spot or more accurately the 'G-
area', and the clitoris, there is very little published information on
other parts of the genitalia which can be stimulated erotically. Most
women regard their genitals as rather mysterious and take the
'would prefer not to know' attitude, he believes. 'Most women have

never seen their genitals – most women hate the idea.' But he says if women and men understood more about what happens, this alone might dramatically improve their sex lives.

In published papers, Dr Levin has listed several 'arousable' areas in the female genitalia. Research suggests that these areas may be inter-connected which might explain why some Sudanese women who have clitorectomies say that later they are still able to achieve orgasm.

the elements involved in physical arousal

stimulation points for good sex

internally
- the G-spot or area
- the urethra
- Halban's fascia*
- cervix
- muscles around the vagina

* *positioned in the space between the bladder and the front wall of the vagina, this area is filled with collagen, elastic and muscle fibre and has a rich blood and nerve supply. Some medical researchers believe this to be the female equivalent of the corpus spongiosum in men. On sexual stimulation this layer engorges with blood suggesting that it is erectile material*

externally
- the clitoris
- the labia
- P-spot or area

the physiological response to sexual arousal
- increased pulse and heart rate
- increased skin temperature
- lubrication of the vagina
- pink flush on the chest
- breast enlargement and nipple erection

Section through female pelvic region

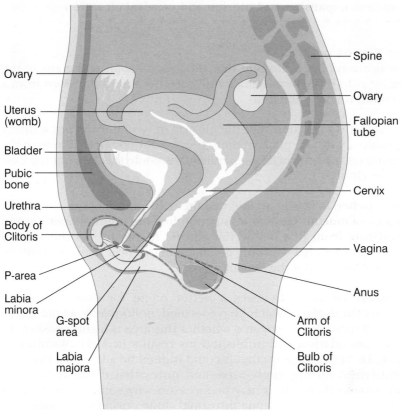

Spine

Ovary

Ovary

Uterus
(womb)

Fallopian
tube

Bladder

Pubic
bone

Cervix

Urethra

Body of
Clitoris

Vagina

P-area

Anus

Labia
minora

G-spot
area

Arm of
Clitoris

Labia
majora

Bulb of
Clitoris

Frontal view of female reproductive organs

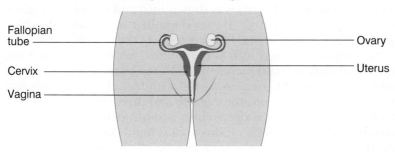

Fallopian
tube

Ovary

Cervix

Uterus

Vagina

- swelling of labia and clitoris
- vaginal expansion and uterine and cervical elevation

●●

the P-spot or area

It was always been thought that the clitoral shaft and glans in the female equals the penile shaft and glans because it develops from a common tissue in the fetus.

In 1987 it was argued that the clitoris in women was not a direct equivalent with the penis in men. It was pointed out that in men the urethra courses through the penile glans while this was not the case for the clitoris.

A researcher, E. Sevely, argued that the real equivalent in women was an area of mucous membrane surrounding the urethral opening and stretching from just below the clitoris to the top of the vaginal opening. This area was only given an anatomical name in 1989 by Sevely who called it the 'female glans'.

However Dr Levin believes a better name for this area is the **periurethral glans** which I have termed, colloquially, as the P-area or the P-spot. He investigated whether this area is highly sensitive to erotic stimulation and published his results in 1991. Within this work, Dr Levin suggests that it could indeed be a key area in erotic stimulation during intercourse and notes that if the area is not stimulated efficiently, it may be a reason why some women never achieve orgasm from 'penile thrusting' alone during intercourse.

Dr Levin made this first published study of the P-area after monitoring whether the area was drawn into and out of the vaginal opening during intercourse. He used explicit sexual videos which graphically portrayed sexual intercourse. As the couple made love and the camera zoomed into the genitalia, he freeze-framed the pictures and took measurements of the P-area by tracing it on the TV monitor. He traced the area on partial withdrawal of the penis and on complete insertion into the vagina, and discovered that usually 50% of the area of tissue is drawn into and out of the vagina during intercourse. He suggests that if this area is highly erotically sensitive it could explain why some women can be stimulated to orgasm by penile thrusting alone, but others who have little erotic sensitivity in this area, perhaps because of a biological problem, would find this less stimulating.

'What is needed is a study of the arousal/erotic sensitivity of this area especially in women who claim to have orgasms from coitus alone compared to those who do not. With such a study we may get an answer to the problem why some women have orgasms at coitus and others don't.'

G-spot or G-area
Another highly erotic zone known as the G-spot is perhaps more accurately described as the G-area, because it is really a region on the anterior vaginal wall which some women find highly sexually arousing. Before arousal the area is the size of a pea but can enlarge considerably.

The area was originally identified in 1950 but did not achieve recognition until the 1980s although it is true to say that not every woman can find this particularly sensitive area. Indeed, while some women find stimulation of this area highly erotic others say it is painful and, when stimulated, can make them feel as though they want to urinate; others feel nothing at all.

The G-spot in the female is analogous to the prostate in a male: cells in the embryo which develop into the prostate in a man remain small and become the G-spot in a woman. (It is interesting to note that some men derive pleasure from stimulation of the prostate gland via the rectum). It has also been suggested that stimulation of the G-spot also produces an analgesic effect which is important during childbirth. It is activated when the pelvic and hypogastric nerves are stimulated by the dilation of the cervix and pressure exerted in the vagina by the emerging foetus (from *Medical Aspects of Human Sexuality*, June 1998, Whipple and Komisaruk).

the urethra
A female sexual organ ?

During research into the Femidom (the female condom) ultrasound imaging confirmed that during intercourse there is a substantial degree of stretching of the front wall of the vagina and the urethra, as the base of the bladder is pushed backwards by the thrusting penis. (It is interesting that in the original work on the G-spot, the scientist Graafenberg, after which it was named, found that the urethra was surrounded by erectile tissue, and during sex this enlarged to such a degree that it could be easily felt in the upper wall of the vagina.)

Dr Levin suggests that the stretching of this tissue releases serotonin from cells in the urethral wall – enhancing pleasurable sensations from the urethra during arousal. His conclusion is that during sex the urethra becomes engorged with blood, becoming a sexual organ which can be stimulated and plays a part in sexual arousal which has not yet been widely recognised.

the clitoris

For many – but not all – women the clitoris heightens sexual feelings during intercourse and contributes to increased vaginal lubrication – making sex easier and more pleasurable. However it is recognised that some women do not get clitoral stimulation during intercourse and some women report that they receive no pleasurable sensation from the clitoris, that it is effectively 'numb' or 'dead'.

So, although the clitoris has long been thought of as the principal key to pleasure for sex for women, it may only be a part of the story. New information has just come to light about its position, function and size. In Australia, urologist Helen O'Connell has stated that the clitoris is about three times the size it is portrayed in *Grays' Anatomy*, the anatomist's bible. The true size of the clitoris has always been hidden away inside women and this new information will be extremely useful for surgeons performing pelvic surgery on women. It should eventually lead to new guidelines to protect the nerves and muscles of the clitoris.

O'Connell became aware as a urology trainee that she had to take special care while removing the prostate in men with prostate cancer to ensure that everything was done to preserve their sexual function. She says she was not aware of any such work for women and in fact found that no one had ever undertaken a detailed investigation of the clitoris and the nerves that supply it. As a result she is now mapping out the nerve and blood pathways to the clitoris.

O'Connell's description of the clitoris is that the external tip connects on the inside to a large, pyramid shaped mass of erectile tissue. The suggestion is that the clitoris is inter-connected with the urethra, the P-spot and the vaginal cavity. The shaft of the clitoris is about as big as the joint of a thumb. This has two arms which flare up backwards into the body. Also extending from the clitoris and filling the space between its arms are two bulbs one on each side of the vaginal cavity.

Most textbooks do not connect these areas together, referring to them as the bulbs of the vestibule. Rather than the clitoris being separate from the urethra, she has found that it is in fact connected on three sides, which adds weight to what previous researchers have already found. This, O'Connell believes, helps to squeeze the urethra shut during intercourse.

Furthermore, the cavernosal nerves thought to control the muscles of the clitoris travel alongside the wall of the urethra, vagina, bladder and urethra.

This knowledge will help women undergoing hysterectomies and operations for incontinence, as more doctors become aware of the exact size and positioning of the clitoris which should eventually lead to more nerve-sparing operations – and save women from sexual dysfunction caused by a loss of sensation in the erectile tissues of the clitoris and urethra.

During sex the clitoris enlarges in both length and diameter: as blood flows into the clitoris the glans clitoris protrudes slightly from the body.

the labia
The labia are folds of skin which contain fatty tissue and a thin layer of smooth muscle – similar to the muscle fibres of the male scrotum. They also contain erogenous tissue that can become engorged, especially the labia minora. During arousal the labia lifts and flattens as it engorges with blood. The direct parallel to the labia is the scrotum of men.

the cervix

Although the cervix has no 'sexual feeling' it may play a part in stimulating other erotically sensitive areas. Dr Levin says: 'When the cervix is jostled by the penis during intercourse some women claim that the rubbing of the uterus (via the cervix against the lining membrane at the peritoneum) gives them pleasurable sexual feelings.' Women who have hysterectomies involving the loss of the cervix do sometimes report a loss or a reduction of sexual feeling.

the vagina

Some women say that pressure on the muscles running around the vagina also gives them a pleasurable feeling.

the vagus or 'wandering' nerve

A fascinating new project at Rutgers University, New Jersey, USA, is investigating which nerve centres become most active during sex by using brain maps which highlight the aroused areas. The work has led the team of Dr Beverly Whipple and Prof. Barry Komisaruk to focus on the role of the vagus nerve which carries sensory messages between the genitals and the brain.

(The word vagus means 'wandering', and the nerve supplies a whole host of organs: it plays a part in digestion, yawning and sneezing and travels through the neck and chest to supply the lungs and heart, among other functions.)

It is understood the vagus nerve provides either an alternative or an additional route into the brain, by-passing the spinal cord, and may explain why some women with spinal cord injuries can experience orgasm, menstrual cramps, or labour pains if they have children.

Whipple and Komisaruk's research proved that women with severe spinal injuries can still enjoy orgasm. How and why will reveal important new information for all women and provide, for the first time, more information about the role of possibly many different nerves which feed signals from the genitals to the brain. This will have repercussions for women who may have an abnormal or damaged nerve pathway and report a loss of sexual drive or loss of sexual feeling.

hope for women with spinal cord injuries

sex can still be enjoyed
Researchers at the Kessler Institute for Rehabilitation in West Orange, New Jersey, conducted a survey into the sexual responses of women with spinal cord injuries. Twenty-five affected women took part in the trial and 52% of them were able to achieve orgasm regardless of the pattern or degree of neurological injury. It was noted that women who achieved the orgasms had a higher sex drives and greater sexual knowledge.
Women involved in another study on the sexual response of women with spinal injuries said they felt a conscious awareness of shutting out sexuality because of their injury – largely because they assumed that sexual pleasure was no longer possible in the absence of genital sensation. They expressed a sense of worthlessness and avoided engaging in sex with partners. However, many found that their sexual interest did return with the support of a communicative, open partner although it may have been a long while after the accident. Research now proves it is possible to resume a sex life with a grave spinal injury which gives hope to affected women.

● ●

One extraordinary finding is that the vagus nerve can in some women, be stimulated from other parts of the body – one woman in the trials experienced an orgasm after applying a vibrator to her neck and shoulders. Their research has also shown that the body releases oxytocin and prolactin during orgasm – oxytocin increases pleasure during sex and promotes nurturing feelings or 'bonding' between sexual partners.

Dr Whipple and Prof. Komisaruk sum up their attitudes to female sexuality with some good advice for both women and doctors on the threshold of achieving greater understanding and acceptance of sexuality and sexual problems.
'Whatever the final outcome in terms of neural pathways

and neurotransmitters involved in sexual response it is important for physicians to be aware of the variety of sexual response that women report and that have been documented in the laboratory.

'It is also important for women to be aware of what is pleasurable to them, to acknowledge this to themselves and then to communicate what they find pleasurable to their partners.

'People need to be encouraged to feel good about the variety of ways they may achieve sexual pleasure without setting up specific goals (e.g. finding the G-spot or experiencing female ejaculation)

'Healthy sexuality begins with acceptance of the self, in addition to an emphasis on the process, rather than only the goals, of sexual interaction.'

From *Medical Aspects of Human Sexuality*, June 1998

• •

the vagina

The vagina connects the womb with the external genital organs and is designed to accommodate an erect penis (as well as an emerging baby's head during childbirth). There are three layers of inter-connected tissues:

● a mucous membrane containing large blood vessels, which is influenced by hormonal changes
● smooth muscle richly supplied with blood vessels which swells upon sexual stimulation and which also contain oestrogen receptor cells
● a fibrous layer consisting of collagen and elastin which provides support but can allow expansion of the vagina during intercourse

Blood supply to the vagina is provided by the internal iliac artery, the uterine artery and the pudendal arteries. Contrary to popular belief, the vagina itself is a poor source of erotic arousal because the inner walls are relatively insensitive to the touch. It may be that the amount of pressure applied is the key.

Light pressure has little or no effect. Deep pressure can be sensuously stimulating if the conditions are right and there is no vaginal dryness and no pain – it may in effect stimulate the erectile tissues of the urethra positioned just behind the vaginal walls (and possibly the P- and G-spot areas). Lubrication is vital for painless intercourse and this depends on how good engorgement of the vagina is – which in turn depends on free unrestricted blood flow.

The lubricant or plasma-like material passes through the tiny blood vessels in the vaginal walls and forms sweat-like droplets on the surface during sexual arousal. Chemical messengers innervate blood vessels, triggering the blood flow into the vagina. The engorgement of the vagina raises the pressure inside the capillaries under the surface of the vaginal walls which allows more of the lubricant to leak through onto the vaginal surface. When sexual stimulation stops, the increased blood flow drops, and the lubricant stops being produced. The excess fluid is reabsorbed by the outer part of the vagina through active sodium reabsorption and osmosis.

how does this happen?
A neurotransmitter called VIP (vasoactive intestinal peptide which is present in nerves that innervate blood vessels in the vaginal wall) is believed to be the principle trigger for the changes in the vagina (blood flow, lubrication) which occur at arousal. Studies have shown that when VIP is injected intravenously or through an injection into the vaginal wall, vaginal blood increases – and so does lubrication – although it seems to have no effect on feelings of sexual arousal.

Note: *work at the **Centre d'Etudes des Dysfonctions Sexuelles** in Lyons, France, reported at the Eighth World Meeting on Impotence Research in Amsterdam in August 1998, shows that clitoral blood flow increases during stimulation of the lower part of the vagina by between 4 and 11 times the pre-stimulation level. The results they suggested, are the same as recorded in the cavernous arteries in men when pressure is applied to the penis. This, the researchers conclude, suggests a sexual synergy between partners in which vascular and muscular responses mirror each other and are reciprocally reinforced during intercourse.*

what can go wrong?

blood flow
With such a mass of erectile tissue it is easy to understand how

important normal blood circulation is to the genitals for the physiological side of sexual arousal to work.

The focus of some clinicians testing anti-impotence drugs for women is to find the causes of restricted blood flow, and the physiological switches for that necessary blood flow. It may be that Viagra-like products may work by improving the blood flow upon sexual stimulation once other psychological barriers to good sex are overcome.

Note: *in men nitric oxide is the key to penile erections – the fuel for sex. At arousal the endothelial cells that line the penis start manufacturing more and more which triggers a muscle relaxing chemical (cGMP) but an enzyme called PDE 5 impedes this process. Viagra works by blocking the PDE5 enzyme allowing blood to flow into the corpus cavernosum of the penis, and an erection to occur. Preliminary studies suggest that nitric oxide is also important in the engorgement of clitoral tissues in women.*

Prof. Irwin Goldstein of Boston University believes a similar process is at work in women: research in animals has shown that if there is arterial insufficiency to the clitoris it can stop the engorgement of erectile tissues thus reducing sexual sensation. It is likely that blood needs to travel unimpeded to the clitoris and all the erectile tissues surrounding the urethra,

Prof. Goldstein and Dr Jennifer Berman, a urologist and director of BU's Women's Sexual Health Clinic which is currently conducting clinical trials, outline their theory that some women can experience sexual dysfunction due to impaired blood flow (published in the *International Journal of Impotence* Research 10, supplement 2, a scientific paper presented to an international conference at Cape Cod, USA on May 30, 1998.)

They identified two distinct syndromes:
- abnormal vaginal engorgement and enlargement required for intercourse. Symptoms: delayed vaginal engorgement, lack of orgasm, or low orgasmic sensation
- clitoral erectile insufficiency syndrome. Symptoms: diminished clitoral sensation and orgasm

They summarise: 'There is a growing body of evidence that women with sexual dysfunction will commonly have physiologic abnormalities such as female sexual dysfunction, due to impaired blood flow, contributing to their overall sexual health problems.'

Pelvic arterial disease may cause arteries to fur up, restricting blood flow to the genitals. Research in America suggests that risk factors for this problem include:
● **high blood pressure**
● **smoking**
● **obesity**
● **coronary artery disease**
● **diabetes**
● **high cholesterol levels**

In May 1999, Dr Berman presented the first findings which indicate that Viagra could be effective in women. She reported the results of the first controlled trial among women to a meeting of the American Urological Association in Dallas. The trial was carried out among 17 women who were either past the menopause or had undergone hysterectomies – over a three-month period one group was given Viagra and the other a placebo. She found that there was increased blood flow to the genital area among the women who took Viagra.

drugs which may influence sexual arousal are:
Antihistamines, antihypertensives, antidepressants, antipsychotics, antioestrogens, central nervous system stimulants, narcotics, and alcohol.

Some drugs prescribed for **depression and high blood pressure** can affect mood and also the blood supply or response of the tissues. A study on the effects of propranol, the commonly prescribed drug for hypertension and angina, in 1990 by Alan Riley, found that it significantly affected sexual arousal in nine healthy young women.

Drugs for depression can also affect women's sexual function – and these include Prozac (fluoxetine), sertraline, and paroxetine from a group of drugs called **selective serotonin reuptake inhibitors** or

SSRIs. Dramatic effects on desire and arousal, and genital numbness has been reported among some women taking SSRIs. One report in the US suggests that 33% of women who use SSRIs will experience a 'loss of libido' and difficulty in achieving orgasm.

The Kinsey Institute in America is currently studying the effects of combined oral contraceptives on mood and sexuality following early trials indicating that some had an adverse effect.

In 1986, a clinical trial suggested that some women's sexual feelings, and the time it takes to reach orgasm, may be affected by **diazepam** (Riley, *Sexual and Marital Therapy*, Vol. 1 No. 1, 1986). One of the women involved in the trial was unable to reach orgasm at all. It is thought that the drug might impair the necessary psychological input required for the feelings of sexual desire.

diseases and disorders which may have an effect upon female sexual arousal

Diabetes is a known cause of impotence in men – and doctors are now looking at the consequences in women. Diabetes affects nerves and blood vessels throughout the body and can affect the circulation of the blood and damage pathways which as we have already seen, play a vital role in sending signals of pleasure from the genitals to the brain. As clitoral insufficiency may be caused by a restricted blood flow it is very possible that a diabetic woman may lose some genital sensation.

Thyroid problems are another cause of loss of sexual desire; either an underactive thyroid (*the condition is called hypothyroidism*) or an overactive thyroid (*hyperthyroidism*) can influence sexual feelings. The thyroid is a vital gland influencing body weight, energy levels, skin condition, mental state, reproductive organs and also sexual functioning.

There are worries that many women with hypothyroidism go undiagnosed because its symptoms of depression, mood swings and muscle weakness, are often confused with other problems such as menopause or even stress. The condition, can, however be diagnosed with a blood test – women over 40 are at greatest risk from thyroid disorders.

Women who have thyroid disease may have a testosterone deficiency – an overactive thyroid increases the amount of sex hormone binding globulin which controls the amount of testosterone available in the body and can lead to a deficiency. Without this vital sex drive fuel you can experience a loss of libido and desire.

In 1987, a study of women having treatment for **high blood pressure** found that 78% had sometimes experienced difficulty in becoming sexually aroused. The hardening of the arteries due to high blood pressure is a progressive problem – more women than ever before are being diagnosed with cardiovascular disease. Oestrogen protects women from heart disease until the menopause – when levels fall women become as susceptible as men to heart disease. In men the same deposits which cause arteries of the heart to fur up also occur in the arteries of the pelvis which supplies the penis. The same problem may apply to a small number of women suffering from heart disease because of a restricted blood supply in the pelvis.

Having **pelvic surgery or radiation therapy** in the pelvic area can sometimes result in vaginal discomfort. Sexual problems are common among women who have had cervical or endometrial surgery.

Hysterectomy will compromise production of oestrogen, progesterone and androgen, which all play a part in sex drive and arousal. There is also very little guidance for surgeons on the nerves which control sexual response. Many women who have had hysterectomies and removal of the cervix do frequently report a reduction in their sexual feelings and response after radical surgery. This often does not show until a year or so after surgery. During the first year women may benefit from the relief of symptoms – such as heavy periods due to fibroids, or freedom from severe and painful periods – and go through a honeymoon period. It is not until later that the long-term effects may be felt.

Some women report that although they do experience orgasms they are not as strong as they were before the operation. This may be due to nerve damage during the operation. There is a growing awareness among surgeons of this side effect, but it is also an issue you may wish to raise before an operation.

influential sex hormones

androgens (testosterone)

Testosterone is produced by women in small amounts and is thought to be a key hormone in sex drive. It makes sense as the tissue of woman's genitals are androgen-dependent. The clitoris, labia probably the P-spot and even pubic hair and nipples are all androgen-dependent. As men mature they lose androgen receptors in the penis, but as women age they don't lose receptors in the clitoris, but levels of testosterone gradually drop: women in their 40s produce roughly half the amount of women in their 20s (**see chapter five: testosterone – the hormone of desire?**). Some women have been helped to regain sensitivity in the genitals by using androgen implants; but it is still considered controversial by some doctors because of possible side-effects.

prolactin and oxytocin

Both these hormones are produced by the pituitary in response to stimulation of the nipples and the genitals. There is a lot of scientific interest in the role of prolactin which has a function in the production of human milk – it is thought that too much of it depresses the sex drive (and it is understood that levels rise at times of stress). This may go some way to explaining why some women get put off sex after childbirth and breast feeding.

oestrogen

Oestrogen is important for maintaining the layer of cells in the lining of the vagina. From the menopause, levels of oestrogen fall: and older women can suffer from a condition known as 'vaginal atrophy' where the lining of the vagina diminishes. With fewer blood vessels supplying the vagina it becomes more difficult to lubricate. However, older women still have the ability to lubricate but may need more stimulation (**see chapter four: sex and the menopause**).

An alternative to HRT may be found in a diet rich in phytoestrogens which have an uncanny ability to mimic natural oestrogen in the body but are only fractionally as potent as the human kind. It is thought that phytoestrogens are able to compete for receptor sites and block the uptake of excess oestrogen and may be able to protect against hormonally induced cancers (**see sex and the menopause**).

progesterone

This is also a sex hormone which balances the effects of oestrogen. Diet, stress, the menopause can all affect progesterone production which in turn can lead to tiredness and decreased libido. Natural progesterone creams which are rubbed into the fatty areas of the body, mimic the effects of progesterone in the body and claims are made that it can help to improve a flagging sex drive .

diagnostic equipment

A breakthrough in research into women's sexual problems has come through an ability to monitor changes in vaginal blood flow, and the development of clinical questionnaires in which women 'self report' their problems.
These machines work in a similar way to biofeedback devices. They are used to monitor changes in the engorgement of the vagina, labia or clitoris with blood (sexual arousal) when women are shown erotic images or are asked to indulge in sexual fantasy, and they 'feed back' information about that woman's physiological state of sexual arousal.
But the problem is that these devices may not be as accurate in a laboratory as they are in a 'real' sexual situation at home, although they will undoubtedly register changes and that may be enough to provide a measure of sexual arousal.
A simple subjective rating scale (when a woman is asked to 'rate' her level of arousal from 1-10) has flaws: women either find it interferes with arousal or the levels may vary from one woman to another.
Sometimes women say they are unable to become aroused – but in fact do. Biofeedback can help teach a woman recognise the signs of arousal. (see chapter eight: adjustments to your sex life)

Equipment used
● Doppler ultra-sonography measures blood speed and movement in the clitoral cavernosal artery and has been used to record changes associated with stimulating the vagina. The study found that blood

velocity increased 11 times that of the pre-stimulation pattern.

- Vaginal photo-plethysmography involves shining an infra-red light into the vaginal tissue and recording the amount reflected back. More infrared light is reflected back to a photosensitive sensor as vaginal engorgement increases. The greater the blood content of the vaginal walls, the more the amount of reflected light.
- Heat wash out or 'vaginal thermal clearance' is a more accurate measurement, which involves a heated electrode held in position within a gold, silver or platinum disc. As blood flow increases due to sexual arousal, more heat is transferred away from the heated device and more electrical power is needed to maintain the electrode at a fixed temperature. Higher amounts of energy indicate higher levels of blood flow and, it is inferred, higher levels of sexual arousal.

● ●

further information and help:
British Diabetic Association
10 Queen Anne Street, London W1M OBD
Tel 0171 323 1531

British Heart Foundation
14 Fitzhardinge Street, London W1 4DH
Tel 0171 935 0185

Sexual and Personal Relationships for Disabled People
286 Camden Road, London N7 OBJ
Tel 0171 607 8851

CHAPTER THREE

sex and the mind

'I cannot separate my sexual being from my emotional being – having a problem with sexual arousal has ruined my marriage. It definitely affects me a great deal because I have very little sexual desire and it is related to pain, making me generally unhappy. It is very hard to have a good relationship with a man when there is no sexual relationship there.' – Eve, aged 27

psycho-sexual therapies

Counselling will help if you have a deep seated psychological or behavioural reason for your sexual difficulties. Counselling won't help if your problem is a physical one which would need addressing first. After treatment you may still require some help from a sex therapist if the biological problem was long-standing and has led to an aversion to sex.

The time is ripe for a complete evaluation of the way psychosexual counselling is offered in the UK and the true benefits. There have been instances where women have become needlessly anxious and concerned through questioning about their childhood sexual experiences when in fact they have been suffering a long-term organic problem (such as a hormonal imbalance) which was causing their sexual difficulty.

This can affect the partner's feelings: if psycho-therapy fails to work he may feel utterly rejected, and it may also result in you feeling desperate because your problem cannot be solved.

Sex therapists are trained counsellors and psychotherapists. Some can undertake medical examinations of women but most cannot. However, if they feel it is the right course of action, they will work in conjunction with a GP or specialist. But according to a survey compiled by Keele University's epidemiology department, very few women with sexual problems had talked to any medically qualified doctor about it.

Dr Kevan Wylie, director of the Porterbrook Clinic in Sheffield, an NHS clinic which has been treating patients with sexual problems for 25 years, says one of the challenges of the future will be separating out women who have sex drive problems (more biologically based) and sexual desire problems (more emotional or psychological) and then treating them accordingly.

At present there are a number of NHS centres able to offer this form of combined approach. There are many more private sex therapists in the UK who operate individually and do not necessarily come under the umbrella of a hospital or medically qualified clinician although they will consult a physician if necessary.

Relate, the marriage guidance charity which has sex therapists in 115 of its 121 national centres, is the country's major provider of sex therapy. A survey carried out in 1996 revealed that around 40% of couples now 'self refer' to Relate. Once again the most common problem among women is 'a general lack of interest'. Some 70% of women with this problem claimed in their survey they were helped by counselling and 48% of women who went through counselling for orgasm problems experienced an improvement.

Sex therapists tend to focus on couples' therapy and sensate focus, a programme of exercises done at home which can uncover deep relationship problems or abnormal feelings about sex. Some therapists will see women, or men alone and work out individual sensate focus programmes for them. Couples' therapy is fine for people who are in long-term relationships and need help but not effective for women whose problems have a biological basis – which may be as many as 30%.

Sex therapy, however, certainly has a place in the treatment of women's sexual problems: an inability to want to participate in sexual intercourse frequently has a psychological cause which can be improved with therapy. But it can only improve your sex life if there are anxieties or worries or misplaced thoughts that need help or correcting. It will also only work if there is still an intact sex drive and a strong wish for an improved sex life.

According to psychologists we are all born with an in-built sensitivity to sexual stimuli – this is our 'arousability' factor. This arousability is influenced by our memories and our experiences, our attraction to our partner and also physiological conditions such as healthy nerves and the right flow of chemicals to transmit sensation to the brain.

This arousability factor inevitably changes as we age and have more experience of life. It is also a mechanism which can be affected by 'over-familiarisation' – in other words having sex with the same person perhaps in the same position in the same situation year after year can be a major passion killer. In addition, relationships change over the years and this can influence how we 'see' our lovers. Partners might become more child-like because of age or ill-health and the relationship might transfer from a sexual one to a nurturing one.

Taking the first step: The hurdle you may face is overcoming embarrassment. Although the taboos for seeking treatment for sexual problems are at last being broken down, it still may not be easy for you to talk about yourself until more clinics become 'women friendly' and are set up especially to help women and their specific and increasing needs.

But bear in mind that professional sex therapists are trained to understand this feeling of embarrassment and will help you. They should make the interview and therapy sessions as comfortable as possible. Be prepared to see two therapists working as a team. The idea is to widen the perspective and some clinics like the idea of one therapist chaperoning another. If you don't want two therapists in on the session, ask whether it is OK to see just one as there are plenty who prefer to operate on their own.

Note: *there is a subtle difference between psychotherapy and sex therapy: sex therapists work on the physical responses as well as the mental responses. Therefore sex therapy is not just 'all talk' – exercises and tasks are set to find out more about the physical blocks and problems, and they can also be used to take the pressure off one or both partners while these problems are explored. A psychotherapist will encourage you to talk more about your problems, and your past which may throw some light on the way you feel.*

the psychological problems

There may be a temporary aversion to sex because of depression, anxiety, anger, miscarriage, overbearing family responsibilities, money worries or bereavement. Or the problem may be more deep rooted and be associated with rape, childhood abuse, parental or religious influences. Growing up in a family with strong sexual taboos can lead to sexual dysfunction, and problems with orgasm. This can lead to feelings of distress because you feel unable to please your partner resulting in a vicious circle of anxiety, decreased lubrication and pain on intercourse leading eventually to sexual avoidance and relationship breakdown. Depression – or drugs given to treat it – may also play a part, along with a loss of self- confidence and self-esteem.

A UK study has found that six per cent of women questioned about their sexual difficulties were depressed. Traditionally women who have lost their confidence or esteem or suffer from depression may be unable to reach orgasm – something 'switches off' before climax, perhaps associated with a fear of letting go and losing control (**see chapter six: the happiness factor**).

These factors can negatively influence the mind which holds the power of an 'override switch' to sex. Negative thoughts, worries and distractions can all bring sexual feelings to a sudden halt. Sex therapy or psychotherapy can help put fears into perspective or even help women change their response – by learning how to exchange negative ideas that sex is bad in some way for more positive thoughts and feelings.

Key psychological problems affecting sexual arousal:

- anxiety
- mood
- anger

the sexual circuitry

What goes on in the mind and in the emotions will strongly influence the 'sexual reflex', say sex therapists. Sexual arousal can be compared to an electrical circuit –

which can be subject to breakdowns, at many different junctions along the route to sexual fulfillment.
The break points are:
- pain – which can cancel out sexual response
- emotional 'interference' with the sexual response such as anxiety or sadness, grief, bereavement, anger
- distraction – fear of pregnancy, negative memories, uncertainty of how to behave. In psycho-speak some women can suffer from 'spectatoring' when you are too busy worrying, and in your mind's eye 'see' or 'watch' what you are doing rather than allowing yourself to be carried along with your sexual feelings to the exclusion of all else

●●●

The impact of loss of sexual feelings

Women whose lives have been blighted by problems with sexual arousal feel guilt, less good about themselves, and experience a sense of their loss at a part of their lives they once enjoyed to the full. The problem not only affects them individually, in the way they feel about themselves, but also others around them, notably husbands and families.

Losing touch with sexuality and sexual feelings can result in stress and tension underscoring much of their lives. 'Sometimes I become angry,' says one woman. 'We have rows about it because my partner thinks that I am 'cold',' says another.

The women quoted here are from Australia, America, UK, Denmark, France and Italy who talked to researchers about their sexual arousal problems for between 40 and 90 minutes. These sexual difficulties were by and large going untreated – even if they had found a clinician they may not have found a workable treatment – and were affecting their overall quality of life. The most common expression was of a loss, something fundamental missing from their lives, or that an important part of themselves as women had somehow disappeared leaving a hole in their lives.

The negative feelings, they said, directly affected relationships around them, inevitably mostly with their husband although some women spoke of their lack of sexual fulfillment as touching other areas of their lives. Several worried that their partners would leave them, others kept quiet about the pain of sex – the bleeding, discomfort and burning sensations caused by a lack of lubrication or inability to become sexually aroused.

'Sex is an important part of our relationship for him – but it was a while before I realised that he felt that way. He suggested that I see someone but I said it was normal, I was just tired and there would be nothing a doctor could do. As a result he feels slightly rejected and sometimes becomes angry,' – Ellen, in her 30s, suffering from arousal disorder and lack of interest.

Living with a husband who does not understand his partner's sexual problems adds tension to a marriage. *'It concerns me because it concerns him – it has really become an issue between us,'* – Geraldine, in her 30s.

'My husband is more aggressive, critical, irritated and unsatisfied with a lot of things especially not getting 'sexually released,' said one woman. Another said her problems had impacted upon her husband's self-respect which resulted in them not being so close as before and with him 'losing his mood' with her problem affecting his sexual desire for her. The loss of sexual desire or ability to become aroused places a huge strain on women, the interviews revealed.

'I couldn't think of having a relationship without a satisfactory sex life – I could not say that to a man: 'you have to be celibate for the rest of your life,' said another.

'To be physical together with a man is very important but I think having an orgasm is not so important. But I couldn't stand it if there was no chance of me getting better,' said Jayne, in her early 30s.

'Sex is very important – but I don't have the desire for it any more,' complained Kate, aged in her 40s. *'It used to be good but now it seems like he is not interested anymore either.'*

'I have put on weight which has affected my self-esteem. I don't feel

so good about myself.'

'I've become passive without feeling – I feel mechanical when having sex, it is not an adventure anymore. I am irritated and frustrated all day and my self-worth and self-acceptance are not good. It is taking up a lot of energy thinking about it and I am not able to feel relaxed in any situation because of it.'

'The physical effect is not there – it makes me worried and upset I have turned to eating more and I have low self-esteem.'

'It worries me that I can't stand the thought of it, it's unnatural.'

'It's beginning to become an issue between us.'

'You try to avoid it (sex) which isn't helping us. Sometimes I try to grin and bear it which is really hard.'

'When he gets uptight I worry that it could be a reason for him leaving – I was hoping that past 50 he would have forgotten about it.'

These heart-rending expressions of unhappiness have not been fully recognised publicly before. Many women reading these extracts will perhaps recognise their own feelings but I hope that this book will show them that there may be a way forward in the very near future. This silent suffering may soon be over, and there will be clinicians, doctors, therapists and possibly treatments available to them soon.

sex therapy explained
Many therapists will include some explanation of the physiology of sex, the body's 'sexual circuitry' involving the mind and the body's responses, and the well-established stages of sexual arousal through to climax and 'afterglow'. The message from sex therapists is that sex does not just involve the genitals but also the mind and the sexual experience may be influenced by a whole host of other things such as early ideas about sex, past sexual traumas, parental influences, and current life stresses. They will also be influenced by what a woman thinks about herself: whether she has recently undergone the menopause (a loss of her 'femininity'), breast surgery, or even

gynaecological procedures. They can all influence body or self-image and consequently have a damaging effect upon sexual response (**see chapter four: sex and the menopause**). Therapists will try to get to the root of the problem by allowing couples or individuals time to talk about their difficulty or even giving them 'permission' to try new sexual techniques or, in the case of an older couple, providing the reassurance that, yes, sex is normal and desirable later in life.

Relate sex therapists, for example, begin all therapy sessions by an intensive assessment which involves an initial interview, history taking and round-table chat. The aim, says Relate, is to 'ensure that those cases which proceed to treatment have a reasonable chance of completion'.

At this stage therapists may suggest other courses of action (such as a physical examination) or the couple may decide the process is not for them.

Margaret Ramage, a sex therapist working privately in central London and also at NHS clinics in Wandsworth and Lambeth, says she always tries to gather as much information as possible, including both family and medical histories. 'Until you ask specifically it does not occur to some women that their hypertension, diabetes or use of alcohol might have an influence on their sexual response.'

therapy
Most therapists believe relationship and sexual problems are linked. Sometimes a sex problem can be based on a misunderstanding or ignorance and can be resolved quickly – but more complex cases involve guilt or anxiety. Sex guilt is a recognised 'condition' and may have its origins in childhood. Affected women may have problems with orgasm and climax.

The objective of the therapist will be to:
● allow 'space' for talking
● set realistic goals for the individual or couple
● encourage more communication and talking about sexual feelings
● provide reassurance
● give permission to try different techniques

- make specific suggestions – introduce the idea of masturbation or fantasy and give 'permission' to participate in these actions
- help couples communicate more easily between each other

Standard sex therapy involves a sensate focus programme designed to identify obstacles fears or feelings through 'homework' tasks. It was originally devised by Masters and Johnson, the pioneers of sex therapy in the 1960s. If the programme is delivered well it can work very successfully. The programme helps couples find out about their bodies – and what they enjoy or dislike – sexually. Sarah Litvinoff says in the *Relate Guide to Sex*, that sensate focus is probably the most intimate thing you can do with a partner – even more so than heat of the moment sex.

Not everyone gets on with sensate focus and some may feel it is too dictatorial, although therapists say couples can benefit if the pressure to perform is taken off. At the start of sensate focus all genital contact is 'banned.'

Stage one: non-sexual touching.
The idea is to help you feel more comfortable with your body and its sensual feelings but take the pressure off performing. You are able to touch any part of your partner's body apart from the genitals or in the case of the man, the woman's breasts. The point of the exercise is to learn to enjoy being touched – or address feelings of dislike. This sort of touching can generate feelings of anger resentment or bitterness: once they are out in the open, confronted and then talked about they can disappear. 'Repressing these feelings gives them power,' says Margaret Ramage. Part of her job, she says, is to give a woman permission to have these feelings when she is touched in a sexual way.

Three sessions a week are recommended although in most people's busy lives this is unrealistic as each session should take an hour or two to work. You are able to touch each other anywhere except the genitals and experiment by touching parts of the body you have not touched before. This stage can include kissing. You will be advised to tell your partner if you don't like something, or use a signal such as touching the hand, and to take it in turns to initiate the sessions.

Stage two: involves more communication, actively telling your partner what you do and don't like. The ban on intercourse remains but by this time you should be getting to understand more about your own erogenous zones and recognising your feelings of pleasure or desire.

Stage three: genital touching with hands or mouth is now permitted, as well as the use of body lotions or gels to help enhance feelings of sensuality.

Stage four: involves intercourse or, in therapy-speak, 'vaginal containment'. This is done very gently without any thrusting, and very slowly, which is important for a woman if she has complained of vaginal pain. This then continues with very gentle movements. 'This stage can be highly pleasurable,' says Margaret Ramage.

She says she has considerable success with sensate focus although she often finds that couples come to her saying 'we gave up and had intercourse anyway'. This result, she says, is a good outcome. Others get stuck for several months between the stages of genital and non-genital touching. Many people need extra help with fantasy or masturbation techniques. A whole programme can take several months to complete.

it may be useful to remember

- sex is a natural response if you let it happen
- try to relax as much as possible
- communicate with your partner if it feels good
- protect yourself from things you don't like by moving the hand away or giving a signal

Note: *it can be really disturbing to discover that you don't fancy your partner any longer. Work with a therapist might also include teaching you how to have sexual thoughts and fantasies and also individual sensate focus exercises which will help you to experiment with your body on your own.*

the sexual response – how psychologists study sexual problems

Psychologists studying female sexual arousal in America and the Netherlands have developed a system which incorporates psychology with physiology. It is called the 'psychophysiological' model and, they say, it can reveal how emotional or past problems can affect the sexual response.

With this form of psychological intervention, women are asked how they perceive their sexual response. This is matched up with what happens to her physiologically using biofeedback equipment. The results can throw light on why a woman might be complaining of a loss of sexual desire.

In a typical session a woman complaining of loss of desire or arousal problems might be asked to indicate her 'awareness' of sexual arousal by her feelings of:

● vaginal pulsing or throbbing
● genital tingling
● vaginal wetness
● increased heart rate
● warmth sensations

In response to an erotic stimulus (watching an erotic video, for example) she might be asked about her feelings of:

● disgust
● anger
● guilt
● anxiety
● enjoyment
● pleasure

A woman who complained of loss of sexual desire might actually have a normal physiological response but somehow their sexual feelings have been transferred to 'guilt', 'anxiety' or disgust, possibly through a past experience. Affected women may benefit from cognitive behaviour therapy which would aim to refocus their sexual feelings in a positive way.

An important finding is that many women do not necessarily take into account what is happening to their genitals – they relate sexual arousal to what is happening externally to stimulate them. This is quite different to what happens with men who seem to need the feeling of an erection. The blood flowing into the penis is crucial for their sexual arousal. It is not until later in the sexual arousal cycle that the physiological arousal of lubrication and genital warmth becomes important for a woman.

surrogate therapy

This is a controversial therapy and only one clinic group in the UK now offers this programme, otherwise known as 'sexual training'. Some traditional counsellors recognise that it may have a place while others remain vehemently opposed on the grounds it can exploit patients and undermine the idea of love and trust in sexual relationship.

Patients are given counselling and exercises to do at home and if they are considered to be suitable candidates can go on and use their new found sexual skills with a training partner – a man especially employed by the clinic – to have sex with female patients under supervision.

Jane and David Brown offer ICASA, Interactive Sexual Training Courses, therapy at three UK clinics. Most 'patients' are men but at the time of writing six women have undergone sexual training with a surrogate sex partner as part of the treatment and more than 40 women have been helped in other ways through counselling and home exercises with their partners.

The therapy was first used by Masters and Johnson in the 1960s at the Sex Therapy Institute of America and was further developed by therapists in the 70s and 80s. Until recently a Birmingham therapist, Dr Martin Cole, also offered sex surrogacy as a therapy and has written numerous papers on the approach.

The private sessions include counselling and teaching clients 'how to free themselves, sexually'. This can include breathing exercises to promote orgasms and learning how to masturbate. After a consultation with a psychologist (who will identify and exclude women he considers to be too emotionally needy or fragile to take part in sex surrogacy) women may be offered sexual technique training with a 'training partner'.

All of the women helped this way have been single, although some had boyfriends. Most of the women have complained of fear of vaginal penetration, or an inability to reach orgasm. In the States where sex surrogacy is more available, patients may complain of negative body image, physical disabilities, confusion about sexual orientation, and lack of sexual and social confidence. Part of the process is learning how to develop healthy relationships, how to touch and receive touch and use communication skills.

One of the women who has been helped was a 35-year-old businesswoman who developed an almost phobic fear of having oral sex with her partner because she was concerned that she would smell unpleasant. She was taught a series of relaxation and breathing exercises and eventually began sessions with a training partner. It took four sessions for her to become relaxed enough to achieve orgasm – as well as bring her training partner to orgasm. When she returned home to her partner 'cured' of her problem, she says she cried tears of relief and joy.

Jane Brown of ICASA says more women are coming forward for help and the main problem is achieving orgasm. 'Some of the women have unexplained pain on intercourse and others find that they reach a cut off point before climax. They are fine during foreplay but then tighten and tense up. Their breathing becomes very shallow and they just seem to stop. Some are fearful because of the way they have been brought up to regard sex as dirty and only for procreation rather than pleasure.'

Many of these women, she says are helped by first being taught how to masturbate – many women never have, she reports, or have never felt the need to. 'But if a woman knows what gives her pleasure, then she will be able to transfer this on to her partner,' says Brown. 'The idea is helping the woman free herself enough to let go.'

If it is thought that a woman may benefit from partner training, there will be a gradual introduction to a trainer – currently ICASA employ two men, (one older and one younger) who themselves went through training because they needed sexual help.

'It will start with relaxation, step by step, so that the woman becomes comfortable with the partner. One session may just involve close hugging or a massage.'

It may take four or five sessions to reach penetrative sex, which is always done under the watchful guiding eye of a co-ordinator: in most cases this is Jane Brown herself.

'We have to make sure a woman is right for this therapy, that she will not become dependent on the training partner or form an emotional attachment.'

Often, says Jane Brown, women with these fundamental sexual difficulties have nowhere to turn. 'Like all things if we are taught something and are then able to put it into practice we learn it a lot more quickly and more easily,' she says.

Note of caution: *always ensure that you use a reputable sex therapist. At present there is no law to stop anyone setting themselves up as a 'sex therapist'. Check credentials and look for a therapist who has been accredited by Relate or the British Association of Sexual and Relationship Therapy. If you are interested in surrogate therapy ensure your therapist does not offer him or herself as the surrogate. This is considered unethical.*

further information
Relate's head office is at: Herbert Gray College, Little Church Street, Rugby CV21 3AP Tel 01788 573241 or look in your local phone directory for a contact number. They will provide you with a contact point for a local sex therapist.

School of Enhanced Sexuality, Top Farm House, Beadlow, near Shefford, Bedfordshire SG17 5PL

BASRT can be contacted at, PO Box 13686, London SW20, 9ZH enclosing an sae.

CHAPTER FOUR
....

sex and the menopause

'When you have gone through the menopause you think that sex isn't a part of life anymore – I sometimes think an older gentleman would take a younger partner because of it. Not having sex . . . makes you feel like less of a person,' – Janet, aged 54. *'I've never really considered myself as getting old and now I can see different things happening to my body. The sex is not as often as it used to be so when we do I use a lubricant. After the lubrication and penetration comes the dryness – it's not a comfortable feeling.'*

At the menopause it may be vital to re-think your sex life and how you approach and view sex in order to find a new sexual balance for the next stage of life which may offer another 30 years of good health. To overcome sexual problems in the period leading up to, during and then after the menopause, couples experiencing problems may need to reassess their sexual relationship, taking into account all the ongoing physical and psychological changes.

Part of the assessment may be sexual style, technique and what you both want from the sexual relationship. Rather than allowing sex to 'go on as before' some radical rethinking may have to be done. But it is not easy, especially if sex has become a 'habit' and a painful one at that. It takes real effort and determination and may possibly need the assistance of a therapist to help see you through.

Relationship problems are common at the time of the menopause. A survey in Italy among 175 women taking HRT found that 27% worried about their sex life and of these 79% experienced a loss of libido and 63% a loss of energy. Some 75% of women involved in the survey were concerned their partner would lose affection for them.

A dry vagina is the most common sexual complaint which is physiologically attributed to falling levels of oestrogen. But a leading Dutch psychologist says hormones alone may not be the cause. A dry vagina could also signal a problem with sexual arousal and stimulation in some women which may need a quite different and more natural approach to rectify.

After years in the same sexual relationship sex may have become boring and predictable – and research has confirmed that this situation can kill passion, effectively damaging a woman's ability to become aroused. Some women welcome the menopause as an excuse to cry off having sex with their partners. But with a more imaginative approach to sex, things might improve – if that is what both partners wish. And some extra help through diet or hormonal treatment might encourage sexual response even more.

According to Dr Alessandra Graziottin, head of the Female Medical Sexology and Gynaecology Centre in Milan, the idea of older people having a sexual relationship is something of a taboo in our youth orientated culture. 'Many cultural and emotional biases still prevent many – from lay people to skilled professionals – considering sexuality as a life-long pleasure and a right of the same importance it has in younger subjects.'

Although all the surveys indicate that sex remains important until our 70s and even 80s doctors rarely raise the topic at consultations with menopausal women.

particular problems of the menopause affecting sexual arousal

- insomnia
- anxiety
- stress
- reduced ability to fantasise and instigate 'mental arousal'
- aversion to physical contact
- numbing or tingling sensations
- self-image; loss of fertility, wrinkles, weight gain and possible reduction in breast size and loss of pubic hair due to androgen depletion

These may be compounded by external problems such as
- health
- retirement prospects

● coping with an unfaithful partner
● depression

physiological changes

The most important change at the menopause is the reduction in levels of oestrogen circulating within the body. But there is also much more awareness now of falling levels of testosterone and how this may have far greater an influence upon older woman's sex drive and response. (**see chapter five: testosterone**)

Before the menopause, the ovaries produce significant amounts of oestrogen as a result of the action of FSH, the follicle stimulating hormone secreted by the pituitary gland. As the menopause approaches, the ovaries become more resistant to the stimulating effect of FSH resulting in oestrogen production falling.

Your body will undergo some radical changes following the drop in oestrogen: in the genital region vaginas shorten and narrow, there is a loss of fat from the labia majora and labia minora and a reduction in the rate of blood flow to the vaginal tissues, the urethra and the base of the bladder. Vaginal lubrication through the cells of the vaginal wall is an oestrogen-dependent process and although this signal of arousal will still happen it may take longer – just like it can take longer for an older man to get an erection. These changes have long been pinpointed as the reason why menopausal women experience painful sex. But there are added factors: for example, your sense of smell and touch may be altered which can influence how you respond to a sexual partner.

psychological influences

New research in Holland suggests that not all women who experience physiological changes as a result of the menopause complain of vaginal dryness, pain on intercourse or lack of sexual desire and arousal.

In fact, older women can lubricate almost as well as young women – the key is *they may take a little longer*. There are many reports of older women in their 70s enjoying sex with their partners without problems.

◆ 69 ◆

Dr Ellen Laan, a psychologist at the Department of Clinical Psychology at the University of Amsterdam, says in some cases there may be other more fundamental and psychological factors which cause a dry vagina and pain on intercourse.

Lubrication is one key element in a woman's enjoyment of sex: without it intercourse can be painful and induce a lasting burning sensation. For good lubrication there must be good sexual stimulation, she says. And that, it seems, is the bottom line. If you are discontented with your partner and don't find him sexually arousing then it may take far longer to become lubricated enough to enjoy pain free sex. A vicious cycle then develops: you may want to avoid sex altogether and give your partner the cold shoulder.

But the good news is that research suggests that new or different types of stimulation will increase the female sexual response in an older woman who is oestrogen deficient. How you might able to apply this in order to enhance your own arousal is explained later in the chapter.

Dr Laan's research has shown that:
● between 5 and 15% of young women also suffer from moderate to severe vaginal dryness – so the problem is not necessarily wholly linked to reduced levels of oestrogen
● women on HRT do not always complain of less vaginal dryness
● women over 50 can lubricate just as well as a younger woman – with the right stimulation

Oestrogen will keep the vagina walls thick and moist, she says, but reduced levels of oestrogen causing a change in the vaginal walls may only accentuate the problem of a lack of arousal (expressed as a dry vagina 'symptom') rather than being the root cause of the problem. 'It may be that an older woman has to try harder or be given more help to be sexually stimulated but it may not be directly linked to falling levels of oestrogen. A younger women may have the advantage of a vaginal wall which is in tip-top condition, but this doesn't mean it is impossible for an older woman.'

These are important findings, she says, because it gives an older woman 'permission' to seek out the right sexual stimulation that meets her needs, which may have changed from when she was a young woman and may have changed from what was desired at the start of her long-term relationship with a partner.

'In conclusion it seems that complaints of vaginal dryness and dyspareunia shouldn't be attributed to oestrogen-related vaginal atrophy associated with the menopause. Rather, vaginal dryness and painful intercourse seem to reflect sexual arousal problems.'

More should be done to focus on the different ways in which a woman becomes aroused, advises Dr Laan. This does not necessarily involve laying the responsibility for good sex at the partner's door, although there is no doubt that partners should be aware of a potential problem and help to find new ways to enjoy sex. But she believes more could also be done to investigate biologically what turns women on and how the brain functions in sexual arousal – and whether there are changes as we age.

*Further information about Dr Ellen Laan's findings can be found in **Hormones and Sexuality post-menopause**, published in the Journal of Psychosomatic Obstetric Gynaecology, Vol. 18, p126-133, 1997.*

Supporting this theory is research in Italy which suggests that a new partner may contribute to an increase in libido, satisfaction, and orgasm in post-menopausal women. But if that is not on the agenda spicing up your own love life with your partner has to be the next best thing.

Couples may need to:
- use more foreplay. Women over 50 do lubricate in response to sexual stimulation, but it just may take a little longer
- use extra stimulants such as books or films
- change the ritual of lovemaking: try making love at different times of the day rather than just before bed when you may feel exhausted. Try to pinpoint when you feel most alert: maybe the mornings or the afternoon followed by a nap

● be aware of all the problems which the menopause can cause physically and sexually. For example, the partners of women with touch impairment need to know that affected women are not shunning them physically but that they need help to overcome a very real and painful problem. (You may benefit from HRT at a cellular level but it may not work on your arousal problem)

● find ways to make sex more interesting – regular sex may reduce vaginal deterioration. Men need to take into account their partner's changing needs and not just assume the same pattern and routine expecting responses to be the same as they were. Slow and steady may be an option rather than the dynamic and thrusting approach.

● find more comfortable positions and ways for lovemaking. Try instilling a calm atmosphere with dimmed lights or drawn curtains.

● introduce some excitement or 'romance'. Women need to be emotionally happy for good sex. Generally, unhappy women have unhappy sex lives. Intimacy is very important and partners may wish to enjoy a closeness without pressure of penetrative sex at every intimate moment.

● be aware of the consequences of changing circumstances: children growing up and leaving home and the impact on stress or ill-health upon a woman's sexual function.

● make an effort to show affection in the form of holding hands, being close and being tender towards each other.

other sexual problems of the menopause

more causes of vaginal dryness
● stress
● excessive douching
● chemotherapy or radiotherapy in the pelvic region
Try:
● oestrogen creams applied locally (with the advice of a doctor) may help improve the condition of the lining of the womb
● KY-jelly is a faithful standby to lubricate the vagina
● Replens is a special moisturiser for the vagina which only needs to be applied three times a week. The gel consist of polycarbophil, a polymer that retains up to 60 times its own weight in moisture. Because of its special delivery system the gel adheres to the

vaginal walls and the moisture contained within it diffuses into vaginal cells
● Use moisturisers and gels during foreplay and encourage your partner to indulge in longer foreplay. Spread the lubricant generously over the labia, clitoris, P-spot, and into the vagina as well as on your partner's penis
● be imaginative with sexual foreplay: a gentle massage with sensuous aromatherapy oils, such as sandalwood, might help

'Sex is very important – the problem is I don't have the desire for it anymore,' – Anna, aged 59.

'I've never really felt he knows truly how to get me to come to climax or arousal. Until recently we haven't been able to have intercourse but have had sexual play. I had my first vaginal repair five years ago having had problems for three years – pain and dryness which has resulted in no sexual intercourse. He had to use a lubricant which took away the spontaneity – and now he can't hold an erection so we are dealing with an ego thing for him,' – Amy, aged 41.

'After the menopause I had vaginal atrophy, there was no lubrication. I still wanted to have sex because I love him and its part of our relationship but then it was bleeding and uncomfortable for several days. There was itching and burning – I didn't want to tell him this because he would have shied away from me a little because it would hurt me. So, I didn't initiate sex because of it. At this stage in my life I could take it or leave it – you need touching and things as you get older, the holding, the sharing of things is important. Over the last seven or eight years we've got a lot closer – we've been married 37 years. If it was just me I'd probably be happy with my life just the way it is but because I also have to consider my partner, it has more meaning,' – Angela, aged 59.

touch impairment

As many as 20% of menopausal women experience such skin sensitivity after the menopause that even a partner's gentle loving touch is painful. Experiencing these levels of pain means that sex is never pleasurable and can become a burden. It can put a strain on a previously loving relationship – it's desperately hard for a woman to admit that she feels pain when her husband, children or grandchildren hold or touch her or that she cannot even bear the touch of clothes upon her skin. This problem has received little attention or medical acknowledgment but it is a distressing condition which may diminish a woman's sexual desire – because the thought of that painful contact is almost too much to contemplate.

Touch impairment is caused by the changing levels of oestrogen at the menopause which affect the nerves. And it may be linked to another common but largely untalked about problem affecting a loss of sensation or feeling of pain in the clitoris. Affected women describe their clitoris as having gone numb or feel that it is 'dead' and unresponsive. One survey suggests one in five menopausal women experience this problem which may be caused by acute nerve impairment as a result of damaged nerves, or reduced blood flow to the genital area.

loss of smell and taste
Falling oestrogen levels can affect the sense of smell by as much as 38% after the menopause. Smell can influence libido, reducing the intensity of sexual desire or arousal and affect the ability to detect pheromones which are excreted from the sweat and sebaceous glands of sexual partners. It can also influence the sense of taste and the production of saliva leading to mouth dryness which may influence how you feel about kissing.

skin problems
The menopause can mean thinning skin, reduced collagen content and a reduction in sebum and release of pheromones. Your skin is one of your sensual organs: if it feels 'different' or thinner it can influence how you view yourself in terms of a sexual partner.

Sally's story
Sally went through the menopause at the age of 40 – she experienced frequent hot flushes and night time sweats – and for the first time in her marriage had to resort to artificial vaginal lubrication. She had always enjoyed making love with her husband and being caressed. But 10 years after the onset of the menopause,

she began to notice she felt 'on edge' when her husband touched her, although she still wanted to make love with him. At first her skin felt over-sensitive to the touch – but soon her husband's caresses actually felt painful. It became so severe that she soon found she was being put off sex.*

Sally first went to her GP with her symptoms – and was referred to a sex therapist. The therapist suggested Sally and her husband try a course of sensate focus – which proved totally unsuccessful. During therapy, Sally's childhood and teenage sexual development were explored and Sally soon gave up. It was simply not working and it seemed to her irrelevant. Sally was referred to a sex therapy clinic – where it was quickly discovered that she was suffering marked changes around her vagina and vulva – and she was immediately put onto HRT. Eight weeks later she noticed an improvement in her pain problem, and by 12 weeks she was again enjoying her husband's touch. She says she is now feeling better than ever and enjoying a full sex life once again.

Prof. Alan Riley who treated Sally says: 'Sally developed a disturbance in her perception of touch which led her to withdrawing from physical contact with her husband. This was diagnosed by the therapist as a sexual phobic aversion. Had this been the correct diagnosis, it was inappropriate for the therapist to embark upon sensate focus.' Sally was oestrogen-deficient and this was evident from the atrophic changes seen in the vulva and vagina. This case illustrates that post-menopausal women with touch impairment can benefit from HRT.

urinary problems
Something like 60% of menopausal women experience urinary problems – and they do affect your sex life. Diminishing oestrogen levels affect the tissues around the base of the bladder and urethra and cause leakage at embarrassing moments. This problem during sex is particularly off-putting, and can be a cause of desire disorders. In a series of 201 women referred to a urodynamic clinic for

* Source: Post-menopausal touch impairment presenting as sexual avoidance: a case report, by Alan J. Riley, *Journal of Sexual and Marital Therapy*, Vol. 4, No. 2, 1989

assessment of urinary symptoms most patients said they avoided sexual intercourse and two-thirds directly attributed sexual avoidance to their urinary problems.

self-image

The transition from fertile to menopausal woman can affect self-perception and self-image, reflecting on your feelings of femininity and sexuality. You may feel 'defeminised' around the time of the menopause contemplating life as an older woman – there is the looming prospect of wrinkles, drier hair and skin, loss of pubic hair and possibly a reduction in breast size, unless you put on weight. (Around the menopause it is common for women to put on weight – maybe up to half a stone. It is a natural way of helping us cope with falling oestrogen levels as we can store oestrogen in fat cells helping us through the withdrawal).

If you feel bad about yourself, 'fat', or mourn the loss of your fertile years – which may coincide with the blossoming of a teenage daughter into a vital, beautiful, and fertile woman – these feelings can directly affect sexual functioning. Add to this the loss of certain 'extras' such as sensitivity of touch and smell and it is understandable why a whole new approach to your life – and your sex life – might be in order. By taking an interest in yourself as an older, wiser woman, taking up exercise which has been shown to improve sexual functioning, and looking at the positives in your life can in the long-term help to turn this around.

During this time of life you may have lost reproductive organs (through hysterectomy) or even body parts (mastectomy) or had cancer treatment (one in 12 women will contract beast cancer, for example). All these issues can influence our image of ourselves as sexual beings: if they are negative images then it will affect our sexual performance. Special help through professional advisers may bolster self-image and esteem and lead to greater understanding that it is acceptance of ourselves and being at peace with our inner selves, which will lead to greatest fulfillment.

A positive self-image is linked to greater feelings of well-being and health and can influence a more positive outlook on life with better adjustment to growing older and less depression.

Viagra for menopausal women?

If Viagra or a similar drug is found to help women it will probably be aimed at older menopausal women initially. It is a safer bet for the manufacturers – because menopausal women don't have babies, therefore reducing the risk of testing the drug with pregnant women. By increasing the blood flow to the clitoris and other genital tissue in response to sensitive sexual stimulation it may be possible to improve orgasm in post-menopausal women. Studies carried out in 1980 showed that after the menopause, blood flow to the clitoris and labia drops. If a drug is found to improve blood flow, then it may contribute to a restoration of sexual desire and enjoyment in women who find sex painful and difficult. But if Dr Laan is correct then Viagra for women could only work once the problem of adequate sexual stimulation is addressed.

New research from the Hanover Medical School in Germany suggests that Viagra might be a useful future treatment for menopausal women – a preliminary study has indicated improved lubrication in a group of post-menopausal women after taking Viagra.

One of the researchers working on the project said she thought women with falling oestrogen levels at the menopause would in the future 'profit from Viagra'. 'It seems younger women have problems of libido rather than of organic problems and so it may be that Viagra will help older menopausal women more.'

Similar reports for another vasoactive agent – phentolamine – found a 'mild positive effect' among six menopausal women with lubrication difficulties. They all received a single dose of 40 mg of the drug and then 20 minutes later watched an erotic film. There was a slight increase in the rate of vaginal blood flow which lasted for about 15 minutes (women taking a placebo drug showed a lower rate of arousal which lasted for less time)

According to the latest research from America older women don't have as many sexual problems as younger women – apart from vaginal dryness. Too many attempts at sex when it is painful can turn into a psychological problem and lead on to an aversion to sex.

If you can't communicate well with your partner this may well be misinterpreted as a lack of interest and lead to a deterioration in your relationship.
With the right help to overcome this problem and maybe address problems of sexual stimulation through inventive foreplay or different lovemaking techniques and some self help measures there is no reason why women can't go on having orgasms and enjoying sex well into their 70s and 80s – just like men – if the desire or drive is there to do so.

There are some 13 million women over the age of 40 in the UK – and it is estimated that one in four women feel the need to try HRT because of symptoms of the menopause. Many women over 50 complain that sex is painful, off-putting and unpleasurable – and blame the menopause for this problem and are encouraged to try HRT. But is this really the answer?

HRT is often promoted by GPs as the menopausal woman's universal panacea – to fight osteoporosis, heart disease, and reduce the other problematic consequences of the menopause such as hot flushes and insomnia – and loss of libido. Many women have anecdotally claimed that HRT can restore their sex lives almost miraculously but research suggests that this effect can wear off after a couple of years. There is some evidence in medical literature to support the idea that HRT can boost sexual desire and that it has a vasoactive effect and enhances blood flow. However, the probability is that HRT or oestrogen replacement has an indirect effect upon libido by helping relieve some of the more distressing or uncomfortable symptoms of menopause. The effect may be only temporary because it is linked with an improvement in the physical problems of a dry vagina.

A survey by Italian sexologist Dr Alessandra Grazziotin found that 41% of women felt HRT improved their physical relationship with their partner.

considerations
The Pennell Initiative has drawn up a detailed report on women's health and says that there are philosophical reasons to be considered before embarking hormone replacement therapy. There is a fear that

the menopause is becoming 'over-medicalised' and treated as a condition rather than a normal life event.

Before embarking on HRT or ART (Androgen Replacement Therapy), which is available in a few specialist clinics as a testosterone implant, you will have to weigh up the pros and cons for your health.

notably for HRT. . .
● side effects
● fear of increased risk of ovarian or breast cancer. In 1997, the Cancer Research Fund reported that there is a slightly increased risk of breast cancer associated with HRT. However when the treatment is stopped the risk is reduced and disappears after about five years.
● coming to terms with taking a drug over a long period of time

. . . and for ART
● risk of masculinisation if testosterone levels are too high
● possible increase in cholesterol levels in susceptible post-menopausal women (an issue still being studied). This could heighten the risk of heart disease.

The Pennell Initiative recommends that at around the age of 50 women might benefit from a health and lifestyle consultation to discuss 'all aspects of the menopause and long-term health'. The Initiative says: 'It is important that women and the men in their lives have information about the menopause and its possible implications for them.'

HRT is not recommended women with a history of
● cancer of the breast, genital tract or other oestrogen-dependent cancers
● vaginal bleeding
● endometriosis
● thrombosis
● cardiac, liver or kidney disease
● migraine (sufferers may experience a recurrence of the problem after taking HRT)
● MS
● fibroids

but HRT and ART may be useful for women
- who have had an early menopause
- who have had a surgical menopause – i.e. a hysterectomy and removal of the ovaries before the natural menopause and complain of loss of sexual desire or arousal
- those at increased risk of osteoporosis

the possible risks of HRT are
- endometrial cancer
- breast cancer – there have been more than 40 studies but no obviously consistent results: some show an increased risk when HRT is used for five years or more
- thrombosis – there may be a slight increase in the risk of thrombosis during the first year of using HRT – it may be particularly high among women with a family history of this problem.

guidelines to a healthy menopause

- **stop smoking**
- **eat a healthy diet rich in fruit and vegetables**
- **try to maintain a healthy weight**
- **increase your exercise – particularly weight-bearing exercise such as walking**
- **have your blood pressure checked**
- **control high cholesterol levels**

phytoestrogens
The new buzz word in nutrition for the over-45s is 'phytoestrogens'. These components of certain common foods, (also known generically as isoflavones) are powerful natural chemicals which have a marked, similar structure to oestrogen but are far less potent. Doctors are expressing some interest but say more research is needed to be confident of their benefits as an alternative to HRT. Phytoestrogens are present in beans and pulses but a herb called red clover (now sold as a food supplement) and soya products contain the highest concentrations.

Research indicates they have the power to block the uptake of excess oestrogen in the body and even raise low levels where necessary and it seems they mimic oestrogen's role in the body competing successfully for receptor sites at the entrance to cells. There is medical interest in their ability to alleviate many common diseases affecting women such as breast cancer, osteoporosis, and heart disease. The effect on vaginal dryness has been more difficult to prove: few studies have shown a significant impact upon vaginal wall improvement. However, they might help contribute to an overall sense of well-being.

genistein
Genistein is the most extensively studied phtyoestrogen and is found only in soya – it was identified as a plant oestrogen in 1966. According to Maryon Stewart writing in her book, *The Phyto Factor* (**see book list, page 125**) genistein has a role in reducing oestrogen withdrawal symptoms at the menopause 'including hot flushes, night sweats, dry vagina and insomnia'.

In 1990, a body of Australian researchers found that a group of women going through the menopause regularly consuming food and drink containing naturally occurring oestrogen brought about the same improved changes to the lining of their vagina as women taking HRT.

In 1992, a study in *The Lancet* concluded that Japanese women do not experience symptoms of the menopause because their diet is rich in plant oestrogens. (For example, the incidence of hot flushes in menopausal women in Europe is between 70 and 80%, 57% in Malaysia and just 18% in China.) Soya is at the centre of the GM (genetically modified) scare – for pure untainted soya, check health food stores and read the labels.

Foods rich in phytoestrogens which may help the symptoms of menopause are:
- golden linseeds which can be sprinkled over cereal in the mornings
- red clover which can be taken as a food supplement
- soya products such as soya milk, soya yoghurt, beans, flour and even cream or cheese

- miso, which is a fermented soya bean paste
- tofu – a textured vegetarian protein used as a meat substitute found by health food stores
- chick peas, lentils, mung beans and aduki beans
- Burgen bread, a soya and linseed loaf available at most big supermarkets

progesterone cream

Trials are underway to test the effectiveness of progesterone cream. Californian doctor and writer Dr John Lee has argued for many years that the falling levels of progesterone rather than oestrogen after the menopause cause so many of the symptoms including loss of libido. He manufactures a natural progesterone cream derived from yams, and like phytoestrogens it mimics progesterone in the body. At present research trials into the effectiveness of progesterone cream are ongoing at the Chelsea and Westminster Hospital. Progesterone cream is only available on prescription.

St. John's Wort

Hypericum is proving to be a very useful herb for treating depression, but a trial in Germany also suggests it can revive sexual interest. A study of 11 women in Germany who experienced a loss of desire at the time of the menopause were given a 12-week course of the herb. Some 60% reported they had regained their libido whilst 80% generally felt better. The WNAS recommend taking 900mgs of hypericum for three months to test the effects.

sensual exercises for older couples

There is still an element of resistance in society to the idea of older couples having sex – and enjoying it. But it is important to recognise that sexuality is natural and normal and can be highly erotic and enjoyable at an older age – although there can be more to sexuality than vaginal intercourse. There are plenty of other possible ways to improve and nurture intimacy and sexual feelings. They can range from holding hands, hugging, caressing or kissing closely to masturbation and oral sex and bring about a sense of closeness even when sex is difficult or painful. Touching, smelling, hearing and visual sensations are all part of sexuality and can be used to help improve feelings of sexual desire.

If you are having difficulty with night sweats and insomnia it might help take pressure off by having one bed for your intimate times and a single bed for sleeping. But strengthening your sexuality through contact is important even when full intercourse is not desirable.

If your children have left home, think about other times for lovemaking: traditionally you may have made love just before bedtime. But as you get older or go through the menopause you may feel exhausted at this time: sex is best when you are relaxed and alert. Try to find some other time during the day. The early afternoon may be great. The message is: ring the changes, it may just help to reawaken your sexual interest.

Talking about fantasies and desires might also help (**see chapter nine: fantasy and lovemaking techniques**) but what is all important is communicating to your partner your needs and desires. Rather than shrugging your partner off, talk about the changes that are happening and different ways in which you can express affection for each other.

Spend plenty of time on foreplay, holding, stroking and caressing each other: slowly but surely rather than 'quickie' sex may suit you better. If you feel a loss of attraction for your partner it may be worth trying psycho-sexual counselling: working out your feelings with a third party can help and can help your partner to understand what might be happening.

Somehow we expect our partners to know telepathically how we are feeling and why, without communicating the facts. If your feelings are out in the open then they can be worked upon, and, hopefully improved. If you or your partner have a chronic physical complaint or condition consider changing your sexual styles or techniques, or maybe investigate different lovemaking positions. Talk to your doctor if you are on anti-depressants or medication for hypertension – certain drugs will affect sexual functioning. You may be anxious about your sexual functioning after having a hernia repair, hysterectomy, or surgery for incontinence or womb prolapse.

Bear in mind that exercise will improve general muscle tone and overall health and feelings of well-being.

If sex is fun for you both, then it can only be doing you good. Laughter is one of nature's greatest healers.

love and old age

Dr Graziottin suggests in a study, *Sexuality and the Elderly,* that some women can experience 'the life surprise' – the gift of having new loves and partners in old age.

'This rejuvenating experience is emotionally rewarding, but may raise new sexual problems particularly if one or both partners had remained alone for years. Also, in these cases, a caring doctor could be precious in treating the problems that could prevent a satisfying intimacy.'

She reports on a woman of 69 who fell in love with a widower aged 73 and attended the clinic to ask 'Doctor, will you help me to be a little bit happy?' She was suffering from vaginismus, reports the doctor, but after behavioural therapy and a course of HRT she went on to experience the first orgasm of her life at the age of 70.

Dr Grazziotin says: 'At the five year follow-up they are one of the happiest couples I know.'

further information:

The Pennell Report on women's health can be obtained from The Pennell Initiative, Health Services Management Unit, University of Manchester, Devonshire House, Precinct Centre, Oxford Road, Manchester M13 9PL Tel 0161 275 2910 .

Alessandra Graziottin's report on *Sexuality in the Elderly* was published for the European Congress on Menopause, ESKA Editions, 1998 pp 513-520

Sexuality and the Menopause by Alan J. Riley, Sexual and Marital Therapy, Vol. 6, No. 2, 1991

CHAPTER FIVE

testosterone – the hormone of desire?

Testosterone is an androgen, the male sex hormone which is also secreted in smaller amounts by the ovaries and adrenal glands in women. It has been nicknamed the fuel of love and the hormone of desire because of its positive influence on the sex drive.

As women age, their levels of testosterone fall considerably. There is a growing body of scientific literature focusing on the role of androgens in maintaining women's health and well-being and increasing recognition of a disorder known as FADS – Female Androgen Deficiency Syndrome. But there are plenty of women who maintain they have had their love lives restored through testosterone implants which gradually secrete the hormone, over several months, into the bloodstream.

At present in the UK, the only licensed testosterone product for women is a 'slow release' implant which is inserted into thighs or buttocks or the lower part of the anterior abdominal wall. The implant 'drip feeds' testosterone into the body for up to a year, although 6-8 months is more usual. At the start of treatment, when the implant is first inserted, levels of testosterone in the body can climb to above the normal female range and with this there is a risk of side effects, increased facial hair, or a rise in lipid levels in the blood which could increase risks of heart disease, acne and greasy skin.

Malcolm Whitehead, a consultant gynaecologist who runs the Menopause Clinic at King's College Hospital in London, is currently working with a pharmaceutical company on validating a questionnaire which will, for the first time, provide clear clinical guidelines for the diagnosis of women who have sexual problems because they are androgen deficient.

With this questionnaire in place, he says, it will be far easier for pharmaceutical companies to apply for and produce appropriate treatments – perhaps in the forms of patches or gels just like oestrogen. This means that androgen therapy could become far more accessible through GPs or family planning clinics – at present only a handful of clinics in the country offer the testosterone implant therapy.

You could in the future have the case of a woman with an oestrogen patch on one buttock and an androgen patch on the other, he said. The problem at the moment is that few gynaecologists are aware of the androgen story in relation to women's sexual dysfunction – and there is at present no easy way for GPs to determine testosterone levels in women. All plasma tests would have to be done by a hospital pathology lab – and it is an expensive process. Malcolm Whitehead's clinic inserts about 20 testosterone implants a week. Women, he says, come back when their implant runs out asking for more because their libido has once again diminished.

Androgen deficiency was originally identified in women who had undergone hysterectomy and removal of the ovaries. But it has been subsequently found that a low dose of testosterone can help improve an ailing sexual drive in both pre- and post-menopausal women, and also treat other conditions such as pre-menstrual tension and importantly, the all-consuming listlessness and fatigue experienced by so many women.

The Jean Haile Foundation, a research institute in Victoria, Australia, is one of the centres leading this work. Dr Susan Davis, the research director who has been treating women with severe loss of sexual feelings with 50mg testosterone implants says she has been getting some 'unbelievable results'. She is regularly sent 'large numbers' of women by GPs and other specialists. Most of the women, she says, have had their ovaries removed but there are others who develop arousal problems after starting on HRT. This is because, she says, HRT can further lower biologically-available testosterone.

Testosterone treatment for women is still considered controversial by some doctors. There are not many controlled studies which show a clear benefit – although there is plenty of positive clinical feedback.

But Dr Davis says it is the dose that is all important: she rarely gives more than 50mg implants. Higher doses could lead to problems. She also closely monitors the woman's levels which provide information for individual management. Dr Davis says: 'I have never seen virilisation in a woman I have treated and I have been giving testosterone for 15 years.'

In the normal course of events, women's androgen levels fall as we age. It does not happen dramatically at the menopause (like oestrogen levels) but instead there is a gradual decline. Its availability in the body is also thought to be influenced by sex hormone-binding globulins – and both aging and the use of the contraceptive pill increases plasma levels of SHBG, reducing the amounts of testosterone available to target tissues.

Dr Davis has concluded that many older women who complain of a lack of sexual drive are in fact suffering from androgen deficiency. In one of her defining studies organised over two years, Dr Davis studied the effects of oestrogen implants upon sexuality. Some implants contained just oestrogen, while others contained a combination of oestrogen and testosterone. The group treated with oestrogen and testosterone experienced a greater improvement in sexuality compared to the oestrogen-only group. Dr. Davis found that this combination also improved libido.

The results of their work, she says, establishes testosterone as having a 'genuine and persistent treatment effect' and she is currently trying to analyse the proportion of women with sexual arousal and desire difficulties who might benefit.

In a report submitted to the *Journal of Impotence Research*, Dr Davis writes: 'In conclusion this study reaffirms that added testosterone enhances sexuality in post-menopausal women and can be of significant benefit for women experiencing low libido despite adequate oestrogen replacement.' Testosterone treatment, says Dr Davis, should be considered for all symptomatic post-menopausal women especially those who have experienced an early menopause.

However the long-term effects of testosterone therapy upon vascular function has not been well-studied in normal healthy women. Dr Davis is now looking at blood vessel function in post-menopausal women who are receiving testosterone replacement implants as part of their normal hormone replacement regimen.

Meanwhile, researchers at Yale University in the US have also found that HRT with added testosterone leads to an improvement in sexual functioning – with notable improvements in sexual desire, fantasy and response and a decrease of painful sex compared to women receiving oestrogen-only hormonal treatment. They also found that vaginal blood flow increased (which physiologically helps with lubrication problems) compared with the oestrogen-only group. In conclusion, the researchers suggest that women who have been on HRT for a year or so (particularly after a hysterectomy) may benefit from ART to help restore feelings of sexual desire.

In a question and answer session at an international conference on impotence problems in Cape Cod, Dr Davis told a discussion panel that there is a pattern among women who complain of sexual dysfunction and who have an androgen deficiency.

'There is a constant repetitive pattern in what these women say. A classic case is a woman who is 35-years-old and has had endometriosis and both ovaries removed. She is on increasing doses of oestrogen but still says 'I feel lousy, I felt flat, I'm tired, I have no sexual desire.' Every woman says the same thing. The non-responders (those who do not respond to ART) do not come out with the same story.'

Dr Davis also highlights other groups of affected women. 'I have seen a number of young girls who have had chemotherapy for adolescent leukemia and women who have had a range of different chemotherapies and say they are sick and tired of being told they are depressed, and tired because of their chemotherapy or because their kids are getting them down or because their marriage might be on the rocks: in fact they have a discrete androgen deficiency. We all have lifestyle stress and pressure but

often you can help these women greatly by simply giving them a little bit of androgen.'
● ●

are you androgen deficient?
Dr Susan Davis says the common symptoms are:
● excessive tiredness – more than you might expect from other contributing factors
● feelings of listlessness
● low sex drive or desire difficulties
● loss of pubic hair
● loss of muscle mass
You are more at risk:
● if you have had your ovaries removed and are being treated with oestrogen – but with no improvement in well-being or libido
● are on the pill
● are menopausal

case history
Until the age of 32, Kate says she never felt any need for a sexual outlet, never experienced sexual daydreams and never recognised sexual arousal. She had a life-long absence of a sex drive.*

When she did have sex with two different boyfriends it was painful, uncomfortable and she only went through the motions because she wanted the companionship rather than to satisfy any sexual need. The first time Kate went to bed with a boyfriend was a disaster: it was simply too painful to consummate the relationship. It took a few drinks before Kate and her first boyfriend felt relaxed enough to try again, and they had to use lubrication jelly. A second relationship five years later was again unsuccessful. It lasted just nine months and although Kate participated in sex (again with the help of extra lubrication) she says she never felt sexually excited.

At 28, Kate went to a sex therapist and was given a series of 'self-pleasuring exercises' to complete. She felt no erotic sensations at all

---

* **Source: Life-long absence of sexual drive in a woman associated with 5-Dihydrotestosterone deficiency, by Alan J. Riley,** *Journal of Sex and Marital Therapy,* Vol 25, pp 73-78, 1999

and thought it all a waste of time. After nine months she stopped seeing her therapist as it was simply not helping. At 32, Kate was referred to the sexual dysfunction clinic at St. George's Hospital in London where an examination revealed that she had a very small clitoris, and labia minor. Tests showed oestrogen and thyroid levels were normal but a further blood test revealed a clue – her testosterone levels were on the low side but more interestingly she also had a very low level of DHT (dihydrotestosterone), an active component of testosterone. It has long been recognised that androgens (the sex hormones which include testosterone) play a major part in the sex drive. But this finding pinpointed a more precise abnormality.

Kate was prescribed a DHT gel which was obtained by her doctor from France where it is used to treat breast enlargement in men. After just eight weeks of treatment Kate experienced for the first time a tingling in her clitoris which had also increased slightly in size. Using self-pleasuring techniques she had been taught earlier, Kate experienced orgasm for the first time. At the age of 32, she now has a boyfriend and is enjoying a normal sexual relationship with him.

Kate is one of 19 women with a complete absence of sex drive who are currently being studied by Prof. Riley. Levels of seven different hormones in these women are being analysed in detail. Kate is the only one to show low level of DHT. Her case is considered very unusual.

Prof. Riley says: 'This case is very important because it shows for the first time that a loss of sex drive has a physical cause. This woman showed a quite dramatic improvement after treatment. However, because only one of the 19 women being studied has shown this abnormal level of DHT the assumption is that it is a cause, but perhaps not a common cause of the problem.'

further information:
Susan Davis MBBS, FRACP PhD
Director of Research,
The Jean Haile Foundation
Victoria, Australia

CHAPTER SIX

the happiness factor

sexual happiness and self-worth

'The great majority of the reason our marriage split up was because our sex life was so unsatisfactory to him,' – Janine, aged 27.

improving your sense of worth and self-esteem

Happiness is a vital key to an improved sex life. Happiness with self, partner, home and work life. The fact that so many women have sexual desire problems indicates that in our modern society there is also a high level of unhappiness. Our sexuality and our happiness are often intertwined, influencing the other parts of our lives.

Can we improve the sexual happiness in our lives? Most of us need some help to balance all the strands of our lives and all the constant juggling we have to face. In doing so, we often forget to take time out for ourselves. But if we neglect our well-being, then other areas of our life will be damaged.

In this chapter, I list some ideas which might help to boost the happiness quota. Combined with other approaches mentioned elsewhere, they will help you create the foundation for a happier, more fulfilled sex life.

They are:
- **diet for sexual health**
- **food supplements and aphrodisiacs to improve libido**
- **exercise techniques to strengthen the pelvic floor and vaginal muscles**
- **stress relief and relaxation techniques**
- **finding out what turns you on**
- **different lovemaking techniques**
- **releasing inhibitions for a more adventurous love life and learning to 'let go'**

diet: *food for love*

The western diet, high in fat and sugar, has been found to lower levels of sex hormone-binding globulin which controls how much oestrogen and testosterone is carried around the body. Good, wholesome and ordinary food – not five-minute wonder diets which make outrageous claims – should be the key to healing your sexual problem. If our bodies become frail due to bad health, sex invariably suffers (although poor health does not always have to mean poor sex). A good wholesome diet will help lay the foundations of good health.

Eating foods like **grains, milk, eggs, lean meat, chicken, nuts, dried fruit, fish, green vegetables and fish** will help boost sex hormone function. Adding foods containing beneficial fatty acids such as those found in mackerel, olive oil and evening primrose oil will also help to improve sex hormone function.

But don't forget the basics: at least five portions of preferably organic fruit and vegetables a day will provide a cornerstone to your health and for older women will provide much of the fibre to help keep arteries clear and in good condition.

Calcium-rich foods such as spinach and figs should be included in the diets of women from the 20s and 30s age groups to help boost supplies of calcium and help to ward off osteoporosis which will affect one in three women over 50.

Some women experience sugar cravings and are literally 'addicted' to sugar-filled foods. Find out if you have this problem, talk it over with a nutritionist. It may be hard to wean yourself off reaching for cakes and biscuits but a starting point is replacing the high sugar, high fat foods with low fat oat bars, or a slice of rye bread and honey. (read *How to Beat the Sugar Craving* by Maryon Stewart, founder of the Women's Nutritional Advisory Service, WNAS). Keep a high sugar, high fat treat until after a wholesome meal.

Bread is a brilliant carbohydrate providing a slow release of energy – there are some wonderful grainy varieties easily available. Try bread made from rye, oats corn and rice to ring the changes from wheat-based products.

Keep coffee and tea to a minimum. Instead opt for camomile or other herbal teas – peppermint is refreshing and fenugreek has a lovely strong flavour, and is also helpful for good digestion.

Eat three good meals a day and snack on dried fruit, seeds and nuts but beware of the calorie load. Cut down on salt which can be detrimental if you are prone to high blood pressure.

Give up animal fats where possible, replacing them with soya oil and olive oil, for cooking. But keep fried or deep-fried foods to a minimum – instead stir fry with a minimum of oil for tasty and nutritious vegetarian dishes.

Much more attention is being paid to the benefits for women of eating foods rich in natural phytoestrogens which may be particularly helpful for women about to go through the menopause (**see chapter four: sex and the menopause**). Soya products are among the richest food products containing isflavones, naturally occurring oestrogen. Soya also contains compounds which may have anti-cancer properties and a role in minimising many of the symptoms associated with the menopause – including dry vaginas. Soya may also offer some protection against the incidence of heart attacks and strokes and furring of the arteries.

For further information about phytoestrogens, contact the WNAS, PO Box 268, Lewes, East Sussex BN7 2QN.

Note: *Maryon Stewart of the WNAS claims nutritional therapy helps 85% to 90% of women revitalise a flagging libido. The WNAS offers a personal dietary programme after a personal evaluation – obtained either through the post or over the phone. Women are asked to list their food and drink intake for a typical week which is analysed at a cost of £48. The WNAS goes on to make up a tailor-made programme. The WNAS has clinics in Sussex and London. For further information, contact: 01273 487366.*

supplements for sex

food supplements
Libido is a commercial product which contains egg extracts which

has been found to improve sex drive in men – trials are planned for women, but anecdotal evidence suggests it works just as well for females.

Ginseng is used in traditional Chinese medicine to enhance stamina and ability to cope with tiredness and stress. It may influence the release of nitric oxide which in men is the triggering factor for the blood flow into the penis. If nitric oxide is proven to have the same action upon the erectile tissue in women, then ginseng will prove to be a beneficial aphrodisiac.

In the meantime it has been shown to boost the immune system, and influence carbohydrate and fat metabolism, and the cardiovascular system. Buy authentic ginseng root for the most beneficial effect. In Chinese medicine, ginseng is seen as a great balancer of the body's needs and is often used to increase the vital energy of the body.

Gingko biloba: there is medical interest in its effectiveness for treating sexual problems caused by taking anti-depressants. A study at the University of California showed that women were more responsive to the 'sexually enhancing' effects of gingko biloba than men. The native plant of the Far East generally had a positive effect upon desire, excitement and orgasm. The US study began when it was noticed that an elderly patient taking gingko biloba for memory loss reported improved erections. The Chinese have been using the plant for thousands of years to treat a number of complaints – it is renowned for its ability to improve circulation.

Wild yam contains phytoestrogens and may help women going through the menopause or those whose sex drive is influenced by low progesterone levels.

L-phenylalanine is an amino acid which is said to promote sexual arousal and may help alleviate depression. The best natural sources are soy, proteins, cheese, almonds, peanuts and sesame seeds but you can find it in 500mg supplement form. It is advised that you take it on an empty stomach and not with protein. People with high blood pressure or who suffer from skin cancer are advised not to take this supplement.

St. John's Wort is the number one prescription herb for depression in Germany, but it is also thought to be a useful benefit for boosting libido especially when it is linked to depression or anxiety.

Black cohosh is a herb which has been studied as an alternative therapy to HRT, and is believed to have a balancing effect upon female sex hormones. It might be helpful if you feel put off sex after having had a baby or at the time of the menopause.

Angelica is packed with plant hormones and in the Far East is a well -known tonic for women. It is supposed to be particularly good taken at the menopause as a sexual stimulant.

Damiana is a herb grown in Mexico where it is traditionally used to boost women's libido. Its botanical name is Turnera aphrodisiac.

vitamins and mineral supplements

Magnesium is required for virtually every chemical process in the body. Stress can deplete magnesium levels – and one of the symptoms of a magnesium deficiency is anxiety. Magnesium is necessary for normal hormonal function in the body – and chronic fatigue is often associated with a deficiency. Good natural sources include chocolate, brewer's yeast, brown rice, soyabeans and wholegrain foods. If you drink lots of tea and coffee it can lead to magnesium deficiency.

Zinc is one of the most important trace minerals and is also required for hormonal function and can influence sexual function: but too much can damage the immune system. A moderate supplement may help boost sex hormone production. Eggs, oysters and seeds all contain zinc.

Vitamin E helps slow the aging process and helps the development and maintenance of nerves and muscles. Dr David Weeks, a neuropsychologist in Edinburgh and the author with Jamie James of *Superyoung – the proven way to stay young forever* suggests that Vitamin E is the most important vitamin supplement of them all. Vitamin E supplement is a good all-rounder – especially if you smoke because you will be more at risk of being deficient in this vitamin.

Aphrodisiacs from the history books

- angelica was used as a potent aphrodisiac in the 18th century
- clove – suggested dose is one or two drops in honey every day
- fennel – a small amount every day drunk as a tea 'improves sex drive'
- ginger – has been used to 'excite the senses' for centuries
- jasmin – Hindus regard this sweet-smelling flower as an aphrodisiac
- chilli – to stimulate the blood circulation

pelvic floor exercises

Many women associate these exercises simply with getting back into shape after childbirth – most post-natal classes advise women to do their 'pelvic floors' to help avoid incontinence. But these beneficial exercises can help to strengthen vaginal muscles enabling them to grip the penis better and to increase stimulation through intercourse. They were devised some 50 years ago by Dr Arnold Kegel.

The pelvic floor consists of several layers of muscles and is a trampoline-like structure of muscle and tissues which supports and holds the organs inside the pelvis.

The main support comes from a pair of muscles which, when contracted pull the rectum, vagina and urethra forward, towards the pubic bone. The muscles form a figure of eight and loop around the vagina and urethra in the front and the rectum at the back. To improve sexual feeling you want to focus particularly on exercising the front part of the muscle which pulls the vagina upwards.

We all use our pelvic floor muscles without thinking too much about them. Because we can't see them like muscles on our arms or legs, they tend to get forgotten, and only appreciated if we have a problem: such as incontinence.

Common symptoms of a weak pelvic floor are:
- you may feel nothing during intercourse
- you may have difficulty retaining a tampon
- you may suffer from involuntary incontinence when you laugh, run or sneeze

One way to identify the muscles is to experiment with them during urination. Stopping the urine mid flow is not something that should be done often, but once or twice will help you to identify the muscles concerned. Another way is to insert one or two fingers into the vagina and contract the muscles – easiest done lying down or standing up in the shower with one foot raised. This also help you become more accustomed and knowledgeable about your body.

Once you have identified the pelvic floor muscles, you can then start using and exercising them. By regularly tightening them for a few seconds and then releasing them you will build up their strength and there are suggestions that it may also improve orgasm ability.

The exercises can be done anywhere at any time. Use triggers such as answering the phone, going upstairs, standing in the bus queue, or switching on the TV or radio.

how to exercise the pelvic floor

Imagine you are riding up in a lift – and as you reach a different level, you tighten and draw up your pelvic floor muscles draw up the muscles a little more without losing any of the tension you have already achieved. Then gradually come down again, controlling the muscle as you do. Try doing 50 a day.
Alternatively, lie down on your back or side with legs apart and chest relaxed. Draw up the pelvic floor – you should feel them tighten and the vagina tighten. Place your hand on the pubic bone and try to tighten the vagina as high as the level of your hand. Hold for a few seconds and relax.

Stress relief and relaxation

As Dr Quirk's interviews with women suggest, tension and stress can infiltrate your life because of a lack of interest in sex and the feelings of guilt and responsibility towards a partner – the feelings of letting yourself down, as well as your man. Stress from work can spill over and linger at home affecting relationships and sex lives. Stress and anxiety can act like a switch – turning off sexual arousal and desire. Learning to relax for sex can be both pleasurable and good for you. The most positive antidote is relaxation.

There are three techniques for relaxation and stress relief which may help you get in the mood for sex
● massage
● aromatherapy
● breathing exercises
But you may equally find that simply having a long soak in the bath, taking time out from family worries and troubles (making time in your diary for a swim or a session in the gym) can be equally beneficial. The key is finding time to wind down, and actively removing yourself for a short period from the source of stress.

massage

Massage is one of the oldest therapies and between lovers can enhance sexuality. Working on your massage techniques with a partner can do wonders for sexual arousal if it is being influenced by stress, worry or anger. Prepare a room with soft lighting, music and good smells from perfumed candles or incense sticks creating a tranquil, calm atmosphere. Ensure the room is warm and comfortable with a soft rug or blanket on the bed, mattress or couch. A back massage will reduce tension in the muscles. Try applying pressure on either side of the spine working down from the neck to the pelvis. Press in with thumbs and then release. After a tension-releasing session using massage oils ask your partner to try stimulating your nipples and genitals in the same gentle way.

aromatherapy

This may be particularly helpful if you are suffering from painful intercourse or vaginismus – and particularly helpful oils are jasmin, to increase feelings of sensuality, and ylang ylang to boost libido. They can be used in a massage but you can also infuse a room with their scent through an aromatherapy vaporiser, or add a few drops to a bath as part of your preparation for sex.

Other beneficial oils: bergamot, angelica and lavender. Some oils are believed to stimulate the release of pheromones and stimulate areas in the brain which promote the ability to let go – so aromatherapy may be useful if you are having difficulty achieving orgasm. Relish the sensuous atmosphere that aromatherapy can bring to a room.

breathing exercises

Learning how to manage your breathing will aid relaxation – correct abdominal breathing can be practiced daily in sessions of 10 or 15 minutes and after a while you will notice an improvement in your well-being. It may help to relax your body before sex, or a gentle hugging session, especially if you think about being warm and comfortable at the same time. Put both hands on the tummy and breathe in slowly through the nose, then let as much air out as possible. Do this several times but ensure that when you breathe, it is your abdomen and not your chest which is moving.

finding out what turns you on

According to new research in Amsterdam we may all be born with an instinctive or innate response to certain stimuli – it may be something as simple as certain rounded shapes.

'We don't yet know, this is just an idea,' says Dr Laan. 'But the important thing that we do know is that the sexual system does needs a stimulus of some kind.' She wants to study our response in the brain to certain stimulating objects in an attempt to define whether some things are more stimulating than others – and what they are. 'I do think that the sexual system is activated as a result of internal and external factors. But sometimes we may not be aware of what that stimulus is.' It is worth people finding out about their own personal triggers, she believes. The advice is 'don't be afraid of fantasy or sexual imagery' if it is something which does turn you on.

Couples in a long-term relationship can get so used to the same stimulus that they no longer get turned on by their partner, which may be why so many older women in long-term relationships complain of a loss of desire or libido, and then blame it all on the menopause. 'It is much easier to think you have a lack of testosterone or you have some kind of disease which is causing this rather than admit that your partner no longer sexually excites you.'

what to do about it
- you could try more adventurous sex with your partner. This takes courage and good communication and it will only work if you are both happy to try
- learn how to fantasise and use sexual imagery (**see chapter nine: fantasy and lovemaking techniques**).

Research by Dr Beverly Whipple has shown:
- that women can experience orgasm through imagery alone
- that their physiological response to orgasm and the 'feeling' of orgasm is the same as that achieved through genital stimulation

learning to let go
'Sex is not the be all and end all for me, but my husband sees it as an equal part of everything else. I may have changed my opinion because of a lack of desire – when things are good I do feel its making a difference, enhances things there is less tension and we are more relaxed. When its good I do enjoy it – it's just (the problem of) getting there.' – Michaela, aged 35.

Women who experience orgasm problems invariably have an inability to let go, to take that extra step and momentarily lose control at orgasm. Relaxation techniques outlined above and in other parts of this book will help, and one of your goals should be reducing tension. But you may also find it helpful to talk over a self-pleasuring programme with a sex therapist.

One of the keys to being able to let go is feeling good about yourself, which may mean coming to terms with imperfections in your body. It can be difficult to change this way of thinking. If you feel bad about your genitals try looking at them in a mirror and do this until you feel comfortable with the way you are.

A therapist will explain that you are fundamentally responsible for your own orgasms – so there is no point blaming your partner. This creates a cycle of anger or dissatisfaction plus feelings of guilt and these emotions are more likely to trigger sexual aversion. You are the one who needs to know what turns you on and what you enjoy, in terms of being touched and caressed.

Sex and poor health – getting over the fears

It is very possible to enjoy sex after a heart attack and after major surgery if the emphasis is on intimacy and gentleness and understanding the partner's needs. Many people who have had heart attacks worry that sex will trigger another one, but the risk is low.

Undergoing a hysterectomy can influence self-esteem but as long as the operation is performed correctly with attention paid to the nerves in the pelvic region a hysterectomy will not take away the ability to enjoy sex. (Talk to your gynaecologist about any concerns) Some women may feel less feminine after hysterectomy and could benefit from counselling (**see chapter three: sex and the mind**). The same feelings may apply if you have had a mastectomy; despite losing a breast or both breasts your confidence at remaining a sexual partner is bound to be affected. You will need to get your fears, worries and feelings out into the open. You will need time to mourn the loss of your breast and your partner may also need help to adjust – don't hide from your partner, he will need to confront the loss.

Arthritis is a crippling and painful condition: and sometimes the drugs given to relieve the problems can affect sexual function. Use heat to relax – warm baths, rest, and massage. You may want to explore different, more comfortable positions for sex to relieve painful areas of the body. Use cushions and soft throws to help make the area for lovemaking more comfortable. Place cushions under the hips and ask your partner to lie in a T-position with his legs across or under you rather than lying with his weight on top of you.

Prolapse of the womb can affect your sex life. You may experience a dragging sensation, discomfort and also embarrassing incontinence. Prolapse can be corrected with surgery which involves taking a tuck in the front and rear walls of the vagina: discuss any worries about the consequences to your sex life – it may actually improve your ability to grip the penis and also help incontinence problems.

CHAPTER SEVEN

looking after yourself

improving your health

It seems only commonsense that sex lives can benefit from general healthy living guidelines. But it is now official: research in the States has found that women with low sexual desire can benefit from exercise – or, indeed, anything which stimulates the sympathetic nervous system, causing an increase in heart rate and blood pressure. Twenty minutes of vigorous exercise can improve the blood flow to the genital region and therefore lubrication – with the most marked effect 15 to 30 minutes after you have finished exercising.

exercise

Less than half of all women over the age of 19 exercise regularly, according to medical researchers. This is despite the fact that exercise can promote an overall sense of well-being, counter stress, reduce the side-effects of the menopause and the risk of the bone crippling disease, osteoporosis. Research has shown that exercise enhances the physiological sexual response, causing a greater flow of blood to the genitals – a vital requirement in the physical arousal process and lubrication of the vagina.

Dr Cindy Meston, a psychologist at the University of Texas, has conducted three studies investigating the effect of stimulating the sympathetic nervous system through exercise before exposure to erotic stimuli. She found that the sexually-driven engorgement of the genitals and blood flow to the vagina is heightened to a greater degree 15 to 30 minutes after exercise – and that this happens in sexually functioning women just as well as it does in those who report low sexual desire problems.

However, there is a quite different result in women who complain of anorgasmia, the failure to attain orgasm. In studies these women show no equivalent increase of blood flow to the genitals after exercise and exposure erotic stimulation.

◆ 102 ◆

Dr Meston's studies suggest for the first time that there is a physiological component to anorgasmia. She says:'Until now it has been assumed that anorgasmia is the result of a number of psychological issues, e.g. religious concerns, fear of losing control, anxiety, relationship issues or a lack of sufficient stimuli or sexual inexperience, that is not knowing 'how to have an orgasm.' My study suggests that in addition, there may be a purely physical element.'

The problems could be related to the functioning of the nervous system or the supply of blood to the genitals and vagina.

important conclusions from this work

● exercise may help your body prepare for sex – especially if you plan to have sex 15 to 30 minutes afterwards
● exercise may particularly help women with sexual desire problems. Stimulation of the sympathetic nervous system which causes your blood pressure to rise, the heart to beat faster and digestive processes to slow down can influence the physiological sexual response in women with sexual desire problems.
● anything that stimulates the sympathetic nervous system may help Dr Meston suggests other things, apart from exercise, could include; an activating movie, watching a comedy, enjoying a roller coaster ride 'and perhaps even a shot of espresso'.

Note: exercise may not do anything to enhance your subjective desire for sex – but it could help your body prepare for sex. The feeling of well-being which results from short bursts of exercise may help prepare you for a loving session especially if you shower and make yourself feel good with some body-pampering products.

Dr Meston noted the improved physiological response after exercise in three sets of trials involving 90 women – but she also found that the women with a heightened response to sexual stimulation after exercise were not aware of what was happening. This failure to recognise what is happening in the genitals (the feelings associated with blood flow to the vagina and clitoris) and linking it with sexual arousal is a common story among sexologists. It poses the question – could women be helped to identify their sexual responses by monitoring them through a small biofeedback machine which would reveal the increased blood flow? At present no such instrument exists for home use.

Dr Meston says affected women would benefit from being taught to associate increases in their sympathetic nervous system with a sexually pleasurable experience by providing them with feedback on their genital responses which shows when the sympathetic nervous system is activated they have a greater sexual response.

Women could then be taught to associate these signals of increases in heart rate and blood pressure with positive thoughts of becoming 'more sexual' as opposed to negative anxiety-related performance thoughts. This might involve teaching women to associate increases in the sympathetic nervous system with a sexually pleasurable experience.

Apart from these findings, which may lead to new treatments for women with low sexual desire, exercise will enhance your overall sense of well-being. When you exercise the body releases endorphins, natural opiate-like substances into the bloodstream which create a sense of mild euphoria. You will sleep better and feel more relaxed generally, and may help if you feel less tense about sex.

Be creative when it comes to exercise: there are plenty of different dance classes to try. A combination of swimming, the gym, an aerobics class and walking will not only help you stay fit but can be fun too. Making time, however, is often difficult. Consider sharing the costs of a personal trainer with a friend or two and start the day early with a workout session. Most swimming pools or health clubs open early for pre-work swims.

Research suggests that post-menopausal women will particularly benefit from exercise – it has been shown to improve mood and decrease stress levels. Stress exacerbates menopausal symptoms so anything you can do to alleviate stress levels may help with hot flushes, and possibly even a dry vagina, especially if you use some of the other self-help ideas found elsewhere in this book in conjunction with an exercise plan.

In trials, pain in intercourse was helped in a group of women who took HRT and exercise rather than just exercise alone. However, if you don't want to take HRT, or you are unable to for health reasons, exercise combined with a good eating plan may help to alleviate other problems, and should certainly encourage you to feel better about yourself and boost your self-esteem. You may then be encouraged to take the next step and address your sexual problems.

There are plenty of other good reasons for exercise: being active benefits the heart by increasing the way oxygen is delivered and used and also helps to keep weight at a reasonable level. An increase in exercise will result in an increase in the number of calories burnt up by the body – the key to an exercise plan is to carry it through consistently. Twice a week every week is far better than five times a week for a month and then nothing for a month.

other health problems

After menopause, women's risk of arterial disease rises as we lose the protective oestrogen factors. A diet high in fat will contribute to arterial disease and the formation of atheroma. In men this can affect arteries which feed the penis and affect erections. Early research suggests that women can also suffer from arterial damage affecting the genital region.

smoking
There is enormous pressure upon people to stop smoking – and although it sounds like a cracked record, giving up really can improve your health. Smoking has a terrible effect upon blood vessels and will contribute to a narrowing of the arteries.

overweight
Being overweight can affect not only your self-esteem and your feelings of sexuality but overweight people are also more likely to suffer from blood vessel disease and be at greater risk of heart disease. Losing weight can improve cholesterol levels in affected women and can help to control high blood pressure. But losing weight takes commitment, determination and motivation. Rather

than dieting religiously you may benefit from reducing your 'fear of food' by eating well, three times a day and concentrating on a good balance of fruit, vegetable, lean protein and complex carbohydrate and less sugary and high fat foods. Women's relationship with food is often associated with emotional peaks and troughs and you may find that there is also a link between food and sex: if you are in control of your diet rather than food having control over you, you may feel better about yourself as a sexual partner. Keeping everything in balance – food, stress levels and the right amount of exercise – can mean lifestyle changes, and even when they are in place don't expect perfection: we all lapse from grace from time to time because it is human nature to want to indulge ourselves.

alcohol

Excessive alcohol can damage nerves in many parts of the body – in men it has been shown to affect nerves to the penis, so there is every reason to assume that women can also lose genital sensation as a result of too much alcoholic drink.

But drinking in moderation may sometimes improve our mood for sex: there is something about a glass of champagne before bed on a special occasion. Drinking in moderation may temporarily alleviate feelings of tension or anxiety – although it can never be the solution to any sexual problem. If you find that you need to drink before sex then you will have to examine why you feel like this, and then consider ways to address the problem.

CHAPTER EIGHT
....
adjustments to your sex life

Sexual problems tend to come in waves and cycles. There are times in our lives when our sexual desire for a partner wanes, or the desire has been switched off because of a partner's potency problems.

The problem with sex is that once you have neglected it for a while you may find it hard to become interested again. This may be a consequence of childbirth. You may have been put off sex at the end of pregnancy because you felt large or uncomfortable. Sometimes it may have been because your partner had an unwarranted fear that he may hurt the baby and your sex life had cooled off or because you are going through a family crisis and cannot contemplate sex. Bereavement, the diagnosis of a serious illness, worries about your child's behaviour, a sick child or a sick partner can all directly influence our sex lives. Sex may become much less of a priority, and if the problem is long-term this can also lead to a long-term lack of interest and a lack of desire which effectively needs to be restored, and gently, compassionately, rekindled when you feel ready.

Many women whose partners had been impotent for years but who have been helped with Viagra or other treatments for erectile dysfunction, have called the Impotence Association helpline, unsure and anxious about coping with a radical change in their sex lives. As a result the association is urging doctors involved in treating impotent men to involve the partner from the beginning.

In this chapter I explore:
● sex after childbirth
● balancing the demands of modern life with sexuality
● sex again after impotency

sex after childbirth
After the baby comes, you may not want sex because you are tired, stressed, emotionally bound-up with the baby with little room for your partner, and you have to cope with an altered body shape.

Research suggests that in many cases it can take women up to a year to return to the level of sexual activity and enjoyment they had before having a baby. And one of the biggest problems is thought to be painful intercourse – around 70% of women are believed to suffer this problem. Painful sex after childbirth is sometimes associated with a psychological barrier after a particularly long or painful birth or one which is very invasive – when a doctor may have used forceps or a woman has undergone vaginal examinations she is not comfortable with.

Changes in sexuality begin long before the birth: as women change shape and become more maternal, there may be mixed feelings towards your own sexuality. After the birth, the new role of 'mother' has to sit comfortably with the part of yourself which is also a 'lover'.

Getting used to your altered body image takes time: you may feel alienated from your body which may be expressed as a lack of sexual interest and need extra help to get over this hurdle. All this can be made worse by overwhelming tiredness and disturbed sleep.

But the change is not purely psychological – there are an array of physiological changes caused by circulating hormones and stretched muscles. The pelvic floor may well be weakened leading to temporary incontinence and there may be pain from episiotomies: both can put women off sex. The pain of vaginal tears can have long-lasting psychological consequences which might need addressing if sex is not resumed within six to eight weeks after the birth.

Research by John Bancroft, now director of the Kinsey Institute in America, found a difference in sexual arousal and interest between breast- and bottle-feeding mothers. A breastfeeding woman whose prolactin levels remain high and whose ovarian function is suppressed has a different hormonal profile to the bottle-feeding mother, he found.

Prolactin inhibits oestrogen production which in turn will affect vaginal lubrication leading to discomfort and pain just as a menopausal woman might experience. It is believed that persistent or long-term breastfeeders may experience a lack of sexual interest and enjoyment and pain on intercourse.

This might be because of:
- greater interruption of sleep
- pain through episiotomies
- low androgen levels
- low oestrogen levels affecting vaginal cells

self-help
- look in a mirror to examine genitals. Scar tissue or tears may not be as bad as you imagined and wounds may be smaller
- don't delay intercourse too long after childbirth – six to eight weeks is about right. On the other hand don't allow your partner to pressurise you into intercourse until you feel you are ready.
- find other loving ways to be intimate – like holding, hugging and touching
- seek specialist help if you think your problem may be linked to post-natal depression
- try and set time aside for your partner. He may feel left out if you become intensely wrapped up in the new baby
- do Kegels exercises to straighten pelvic floor (see page 97)
- ensure you and your partner enjoy some form of relaxation therapy together (**see chapter six: the happiness factor**)
- alternatively , try the 'stimulation therapy' mentioned on page 103 – you could find that an exciting video may do the trick and provide the right physiological starting point for sex

Sheila Kitzinger summed up some of the problems in her book, *Woman's Experience of Sex* (Penguin).
'When the birth has been difficult she may be really frightened of and alienated from her body and alarmed by the changes that have been forced on it.'I felt I might tear at any moment', 'after the poking and prodding I wanted time to recover and have my body to myself again'. She wonders whether she will ever be able to feel that it is hers again to experience with sexual delight. She may be bruised, and sore, and when she shifts from one buttock to the other the stitches in her perineum make her think she is sitting on embedded thorns or slivers of glass.'

A high-tech labour may influence how you feel about your body after birth; if all control is taken from you, you may feel alienated from your body and need help to restore your confidence in it, and to be able to draw pleasure from it. There are fears to overcome: after the delivery; some women shy away from their partner's sexual advances because they associate vagina with birth rather than vagina with pleasure.

lovemaking after the birth

The perineum may be very sensitive and sore after birth especially with an episiotomy. Talk to your midwife beforehand about your thoughts on episiotomy versus a tear. Sometimes tears can painful.

- use a gel moisturising lotion to help smooth the way for more comfortable intercourse
- place your hips on cushions so that there is no pressure on your back; you may be more comfortable on top – you have more control over penetration this way
- if you have had a Caesarean section it will be important for your partner not to press down on the scar. Use positions where this is avoided such as rear entry intercourse or lying together in a spoons position.
- if you are breast feeding ask your partner not to put much pressure on your breasts. Some women have problems coming to terms with their breasts as sexually stimulating while they are breast feeding. This is quite normal but you will need to discuss your feelings with your partner.
- explore the vaginal area yourself before you embark on intercourse to find out what feels comfortable and what feels sore. Communicate this to your partner

Sheila Kitzinger suggests this lovemaking technique

'Fear that you are going to have pain is very likely to make you tense up inside which then causes a constriction which causes you further pain. So it is important to be able to release your pelvic floor muscles and make them soft loose and velvety as your partner comes in. Some men think the only way to penetrate is to push. This is not so. If a man has a strong erection he should be able to wait at

the entrance to the vagina (with) only the tip of his penis
between the outer folds of your labia and you come down
to meet him with your muscles. You will discover when
you have bulged the muscles out you can then make little
movements with them, alternately contracting and
releasing so that you stroke him lightly. He avoids all
thrusting and leaves the action to you.'

● ●

resuming sex with an impotent man

If your partner has had problems with erectile dysfunction, but has
had his potency restored with drugs or one of the other treatments
now available, the new and possibly high demands for sex may be of
particular concern. His potency may have been restored without you
knowing about it and without your opinion being sought: doctors
report that men frequently come alone to impotence clinics and
exclude their partners. One sex therapist said she knew of marriages
which have broken up following the prescription of Viagra.

After months or possibly even years of living with impotence, it can
take a great deal of adjustment to cope with sex again on a far more
regular basis than you have may have been used to for a long time.
During that time your body may have changed (see **chapter four:
sex and the menopause**) and you may need extra help and
stimulation from your partner to get you in the mood for sex.
However, facing a re-launch of your sex life can be worrying and off
putting and may not even be desired. But if you bottle up your
feelings believing yourself to be selfish or cold-hearted if you do not
succumb to sex, this can lead to problems with vaginal dryness or
other physical problems associated with anxiety and lack of desire
or sex drive. It becomes a vicious circle: dread or fear of sex,
deterioration of relationship, and eventually a possibly breakdown
in the partnership.

So much has been written about how great it is for men to have their
potency restored with the new impotence treatments which include
injections, pumps and tablets. It is thought that between 70 and 90%
of men affected by erectile dysfunction can be helped. But there is
concern that little thought has been given to the women who may
have not had sex with their partner for years.

'Suddenly some women are being faced with an erection after 10 or 15 years without sex,' says Victoria Lehman, a sex therapist with the Impotence Association. 'And it can be quite worrying.' The association would like to see more doctors involving female partners in erectile dysfunction consultations, so that the woman's perspective on the new situation can be openly expressed, allowing any fears and anxieties to be taken into account. Victoria says at present many men seek treatment alone, and sometimes without telling their partner. This could cause great problems within a relationship.

'A woman can face many concerns. Such as if he can do this with me he can do this now with someone else? There may be fears of pregnancy and also of pain on intercourse. After years of not having sex a woman may find it uncomfortable especially if she has experienced thinning of the vaginal walls. How can a woman say no comfortably to a partner who has had his potency restored? These issues have not been addressed and they are causing women anxiety.'

Women may have fallen into a comfortable way of life with an impotent man, still enjoying intimacy, cuddles or even orgasm without penetrative sex. Getting used to demands for penetrative sex and possibly frequent demands, can be unwelcome for some, says Victoria. Ideally there needs to be communication between the couple, and some discussion of the potential problems with the prescribing doctor. 'A lot of women have not had sex for many years in this situation and it can all be a bit of a shock after 20 years – we need doctors, and their patients, to open their eyes to this,' she adds.

A woman may have added problems such as fears of losing her newly potent partner, fears that he may not fancy her sexually any more, and even worries that they might die as a result of taking Viagra. 'It is so important to talk to women rather than assume that they feel good about their partners having erections again.'

balancing sexuality with modern life
Modern women are faced with more roles and responsibilities than ever before. Women have fought long and hard for equality but in the 'real world' it frequently feels as though everything is horribly out of balance. Not only are we pursuing careers, but also nurturing

children and trying to be a responsible parent with time to give, for listening, playing, help and guiding! Even if you buy in help such as a nanny or au pair you are still needed to be available as a taxi driver to children's numerous social events, and be around when a child is sick. There may be extra responsibilities such as looking after an aging or dying parent or helping out with a partner's problems. You have to fit in time for exercise, shopping, and spending time with friends. You are probably coping with this huge load without the back up of an extended family. Today we frequently live away from our families and don't have a network of support.

All these demands pressurise our time and sap our energy levels. Sometimes a partner reaching out expecting sex last thing at night is simply the last straw. You feel you have given out all day long and just want some time to yourself, albeit five minutes before sleep takes over. At these times sex becomes much less of a priority, especially if you normally have sex at bedtime.

Scientists in Quebec have confirmed that career women who juggle difficult jobs with the demands of a family face greater risk of stress-related illnesses than their male partners. These women were more likely to have high blood pressure if they had at least two children

A frantic, busy life can only benefit from some radical reappraisal. You may need to ask your partner to help share the load, or encourage teenage children to take more responsibility for themselves. Adapting and changing to suit the situation is something we do in other areas of life when we change jobs or retire. Why not adapt and change in just the same way with a commitment to an improved sex life? We probably don't because most of us find it hard to discuss our problems openly. It takes courage to address this area of life but if you can summon it, the rewards will be great.

The starting point is finding more time for your partner. The next step is understanding how your sex lives might have changed from the first flush of romance and especially after having children. 'Sex at 40 will be different from sex at 20,' says Victoria Lehman. 'What relationships under pressure might benefit from is a change in attitude.'

Focusing on the importance of intimacy, ensuring you spend time alone together, and understanding the health-giving benefits of a fulfilling and regular sex life (physically and mentally) are all important. Sex doesn't always have to be a long drawn out process: a 'quickie' can be just as stimulating – as long as you are both aroused enough to participate fully. Sex can actually relieve some of the pressure we are under; it has been shown to reduce stress levels and reduce anxiety. Sex triggers hormones which encourage a closer bonding with our partner.

'The problem is that we all have high standards and expectations. If something is broken we won't hang around, we'll leave the situation or move on,' says Victoria Lehman.

Finding time for intimacy is your key to improved sexuality and it is possible to work into a busy schedule: it is making the commitment to do it. It may only need some small, simple actions like switching off the TV and going to bed with each other instead. Or making space in your diary to spend the time with a partner rather than rushing off to the gym or to your separate leisure activities. By working on maintaining the central relationship in your life and not allowing it to drift because you are under pressure, you may find that an improved sex life follows quite naturally. But it may take planning, care, and nurturing. Above all it takes commitment from each other to make things better.

CHAPTER NINE
....
fantasy and lovemaking techniques

In the second chapter (sex and physiology) the known areas providing sexual pleasure are listed. If your sex life is proving less than satisfactory you may want to experiment with new sexual positions to stimulate these areas. This may involve your partner penetrating from a different angle, or gently stimulating your P-spot or G-spot during foreplay. Every woman is individual and you also need to know what stimulates you – and then have the courage to talk it through with your partner.

Talking about sexual response involves honesty and trust: it gets easier after the first attempts. Many women find they don't have the words: use your own words and private signals to express how you feel and what pleases you sexually: this alone can really help to develop a bond.

● learn about what pleases you, rather than go along with what you have always done. Masturbation and self-pleasuring may not appeal to everyone but many sex therapists recommend it as a way of discovering what arouses you as an individual
● examine psychological 'blocks'. Prof. Riley believes that women are governed far more by psychological influences than men. Any conflict can immediately block arousal. If you are stressed or have had a bad day or feel angry and upset at your partner, your feelings will influence your sexual arousal in the evening. If, on the other hand you have had a good, fulfilling and satisfactory day you will be far more in the mood for love
● many women experience 'reflected desire', they get turned on by their partner's desire for them. US researchers have found that women respond to being desired and thought of as attractive and sexy – and then being told about it. Encourage compliments from your partner and explain you need to 'feel loved' and admired
● consider your sexual compatibility. Some women who think they have no sex drive may in fact simply have a low sex drive which is

normal for them. But this sex drive may become 'suffocated' by a partner who wants sex more often than his partner. One way to find out is to abstain from sex for one or two weeks: but keep a diary on when you feel sexy and when your partner does. It may be that with the pressure for sex off for a fortnight by day 12 you may be feeling very sexy.

Then it is a matter of compromise: once your partner understands your sex drive and you understand his you should strive to find a middle course so that you are both satisfied and the pressure for sex is removed.

- over familiarisation can be a passion killer. Long-term-relationships become flooded with 'non sexual concerns' which wipe out the sexual spark. Ensure you each have your own space and respect your time alone, making times spent together special.

This is much harder for couples who work and live together but it is something worth considering if you find you lack the desire you once had for each other. You will need to work out how to get around this on your own terms in a way to suit you both. Try to vary the time and place you make love rather than the same night, the same time and in the same position

- consider viewing some sexy movies together. Some companies now make videos specifically for women, by women. These erotic films are often used therapeutically by sex clinics who want to study arousal problems. (Although not an erotic video as such, you might find it useful to watch *A Woman's Guide to Loving Sex*, a companion video to the book of the same name by Tricia Barnes and Lee Rodwell, Boxtree, £12.99.)The video is produced by Chrysalis Home Video. Or write to Bluemoon Films at 89 London Lane, Bromley, Kent for their video list, which includes *The Secrets of Sacred Sex*, and *Celebrating Orgasm* with Betty Dodson the author of *Sex for One*. This includes suggestions for clitoral stimulation and women talking about the benefits of sexuality sessions through 'increased self-knowledge, greater self-esteem and enhanced partner relationships.'

- if films are not your scene try reading some arousing books just before bed. Women's top shelf books are growing in popularity and are very easy to get hold of. Women often find they are turned on by words in a book followed by advances from their partner.

- take time to ask your partners about their likes and dislikes. Be interested as well as interesting; this helps build a satisfying and fulfilling relationships. Most people find that sex is really fulfilling when there is trust and communication and a sense of contentment with each other.
- use your friends as a sounding board: girlie nights talking about sex problems can be really therapeutic and are a useful time to offload. Your problems may not seem so frightening when you hear about what others are going through. Friends like to talk about their sexuality and sensuality – use this positive outlet.
- try to become more 'pleasure orientated' rather than 'goal orientated'. Don't just assume that sexual activity has to end in penetrative sex and orgasm. This puts pressure on you and your partner to perform. Rather, view each aspect of intimacy such as kissing or holding as an entity in its own right not necessarily leading on to any 'next stage'.

Fantasy is an important part of a sex life: but some women maintain they cannot and do not fantasise at all. In one survey only 50% of women said they fantasise while making love. Don't be put off by the word' fantasy'. If you can day dream then you can fantasise.

Betty Dodson says in her book *Sex for One* it had never dawned on her to use her mind for sexual content until she was 36-years-old: when a lover began to arouse her with his sexual fantasies, fuelled by his imagination. Dodson says she began to develop and expand her fantasy world by replaying a 'hot sexual experience'. Sometimes it was a recent experience and sometimes she would change a few details. But it was reading books and magazines which helped her most. However, she also discovered that simply looking at attractive men in a magazine did not do the trick: she says she needed some kind of emotional or intellectual interaction to inspire the desire.

In her book she lists the sexual fantasy scenarios which are most popular. These include
- playing doctor
- being made to perform sexually against your will
- being punished or humiliated
- getting strip searched
- having sex with a football team or other 'gang bang' scenes

There is no certification of fantasies: they can be as far fetched as you like. Research has shown that women's fantasies change with the times. Whereas women once fantasised about being raped – today it is more likely that women fantasise about overpowering a man. Experts in the field of sexual fantasy say that women have changed from the submissive role in their fantasies – to a more dominant one.

You can find out more information about fantasies by reading the books of American author Nancy Friday. She wrote *My Secret Garden* in 1974 and it lists the fantasies of many women – from rape scenes to those involving submission or humiliation. Her later books written in the 1990s shows how women's fantasies have moved on – women have become more empowered in their lives and also in their sexual thoughts and daydreams.

Some women find classic romantic notions are the greatest turn on – think of the numbers of Mills and Boon books which are still read by millions of women. But once again story lines have changed. Rather than women being seen as being seduced they are now the ones to remove the men's clothing, to take control, active rather than passive active in their sexual fantasy

However acting on a fantasy can require the permission of a participating partner. Fantasising about bondage or seducing a man is fine, but if you actually use any of these techniques then you must also have an escape route – a way out. Try using code words or signals which mean 'that's enough'. It keeps this type of sexual activity safe as well as keeping the lines of communication and reality open.

Fantasies allow people to experience situations and pleasures they normally may not find accessible or which may not be socially acceptable. They can help prepare you for sexual intercourse with your partner by using the imagination to help with the sexual arousal process. Mentally rehearsing sexual situations without guilt may pave the way for an improved sexual response and improved sexual feelings particularly if your problem is one of slow arousal – or you are able to become sexually aroused, but it takes time.

Useful aids
● *My Secret Garden: Women's Sexual Fantasies*, Pocket Books, 1974

● Look out for films by Candida Royalle. She founded Femme
Productions in 1984 in order to create erotic films from a
woman's perspective that could be enjoyed by both women
and men. She has made at least 14 films. The Femme line has
gone on to win several awards and is now distributed worldwide
by Adam & Eve.

The Internet has spawned cyber fantasy land: there are interactive
online chat rooms in which participants can write out their wildest
fantasies without anyone knowing them – or their gender. Fantasies
are portrayed in books and films written and produced especially
for women and these may help you develop fantasies of your own.

In summary, fantasies reveal what it is that you personally find
arousing. You can begin to learn how to fantasise by simply thinking
of erotic images and then start to talk about them with your partner.
You could ask your partner to reciprocate or encourage him to speak
to you in detail about them: he may prefer to do this with the lights
dimmed or off, and you lying next to him listening and eventually
responding.

kissing
In long-term relationships kissing is often forgotten: but men and
women do find deep prolonged kissing stimulating. Try and recall
the early days of your romance and how you enjoyed kissing. Try
using it earlier in the day as a signal or prelude to the promise of sex
in the evening. Tell your partner where you enjoy being kissed:
experiment with different parts of the body, the back, neck, ears,
even the feet and toes.

lots of foreplay
Women who suffer low sexual desire might find it helpful to
concentrate on long bouts of foreplay with a partner; many women
can reach orgasm with foreplay alone. Ask your partner to take time
to explore your external genitalia rather than simply focusing on
penetrating the vagina; that, as you will have read earlier, may not
be enough to excite you sexually – other surfaces need to be
explored, touched, rubbed and caressed and these are detailed in
the earlier chapter.

Take some pressure off lovemaking sessions by agreeing with your partner that full intercourse need not happen every time you become intimate. Just lying with your partner, stroking, each other, talking, hugging and kissing each other can sometimes be enough – tension and tightness of the vagina can happen when there is pressure to perform or take part in vaginal intercourse without the necessary preparation.

Ensure the room is ready for love; with soft lights, aromatherapy vaporiser burning, soft music, plenty of cushions, rugs and covers. Concentrate solely on your partner: clear all thoughts of children and work from your mind.

Foreplay can include undressing each other, touching each other in the genital area and all over the body, kissing, oral sex, – gentleness and lightness of touch should be the key words at this stage. This approach will help to relax you and also helps you to enjoy feeling wanted and desired without the pressure of full, thrusting and possibly painful intercourse. After prolonged foreplay you may feel lubricated enough to want to make love and you may then be ready for more dynamic thrusting.

masturbation – or 'self-loving'
You are unlikely to have an orgasm if you have negative feelings about your partner – anger, sadness, bitterness. These conflicts may need to be resolved before you can let go again with your partner.

The next step is discovering what turns you on: you may need to learn how to masturbate and a good therapist will provide you with information about how to do this if you have never masturbated before.

You will be reassured that it is not 'dirty' or 'abnormal' and you may need this reassurance if you were discouraged from touching yourself as a child. Some women find this idea distasteful or embarrassing to discuss but remember that your genitals belong to you. Your partner will not magically or telepathically know what to do but if you explore yourself and find out what is pleasurable you will be able to communicate this to him later. You need to know what turns you on in order to tell your partner. Ensure you have your own space and private time to explore your body. Some women masturbate regularly and climax without the distractions of a partner. This is entirely normal. Some therapists recommend sexual fantasising to help women masturbate and reach a climax.

Such women are usually anxious, have low self-esteem, feel unloved or have a fear of rejection. Try some of the suggestions above but remember that open communication with your partner which includes explaining just how you feel, and what you like during sex, will help to improve your sexual relationship and fulfillment. It does take courage, especially if you have been unable to talk openly before and you may need specialist help to see you through until you gain confidence.

John Bancroft in his book *Human Sexuality and Its Problems* explains that you will benefit from indulging in some healthy pampering, listening to good music, reading interesting, erotic literature, looking at pictures and enjoying nice smells.

In a self-exploration programme you will be encouraged to explore your own genitalia – using a mirror. It is surprising how little women know about their own genitals or prefer not to know. Self-exploration can lead on to gentle genital caressing – fears of loss of control and of masturbation may appear at this stage – but it provides an opportunity to identify the time these feelings appear which can be talked about later with a therapist or your partner.

tips

- ask your partner to tell you what he likes and loves about you
- if it helps, have a glass of wine before lovemaking. Take care, however, as too much will adversely affect your ability to make love
- learn to become more intimate with your partner. Talk more to each other, kiss, hold, touch and hug each other and confide your fears more to each other. Sex promotes the release of oxytocin, a chemical which helps bonding between sexual partners

Masturbation is all about knowing yourself – and discovering what gives you pleasure. If you don't know then you can't tell a partner. This can lead to unsatisfactory sex or a loss of desire for sex. Many women do feel uncomfortable about self-discovery or self-pleasuring. You may feel embarrassed or perfectly silly: but take your time and you may find it very instructive and helpful. It may help to watch a sexy video or read a book first or during masturbation.

Start by stroking the genitals and gently touching the clitoris, discovering its position. You may find a little lubrication helps. Concentrate on stimulating rather than rubbing the clitoris – rubbing can actually be quite painful. Slip a finger inside the vagina and see if you enjoy the sensation from different angles. You may find some sensitive or dry areas you could tell your partner about.

Inside the vagina between the urethra and front wall of the vagina is the G-spot: but don't worry if you can't feel anything. Not every woman can. You may want to try bringing yourself to orgasm, possibly using fantasy.

Sexual techniques

changing positions

Finding out what pleases you should be fun – and exciting. But you will need to be able to talk to your partner and be willing to try different techniques with the aim of restoring sexual dynamism in your relationship. This might be difficult at first but keep trying – it really could help to improve the quality of your sex life.

Changing your lovemaking positions may be the trigger to improving your desire if your problem is one of a long-term relationship and fading libido. You may find that your erogenous zones are not being aroused – they are being ignored. You may have become quite bored with the routine of being on top or underneath. The missionary position with the woman underneath and the man on top can make you feel trapped or squashed, although it is ideal for kissing and talking to each other. This position may not be ideal for stimulation of the G-spot or the P-spot. You can ring the changes by wrapping legs around your partner's waist or even over his shoulders.

For deeper penetration in the missionary position, pull your knees right up to your chest then place your legs over your partner's back so that the penis jostles against the enlarged urethra. You may have to move about quite considerably to find the 'right' position in which you enjoy the best stimulation.

Alternatively, sit upright and astride your partner, or sit up facing each other. Being on top can be erotic for women and with greater freedom of movement than lying underneath the partner. Use the techniques outlined above of fantasy and masturbation. Take control by moving your partner's hand into the most arousing position.

Many women say that being on top is more stimulating: because they are able to control the amount of clitoral stimulation more accurately. Strategically place pillows under hips to raise the genital area for a different form of sensation. Lying face to face is another gentle way of making love. – it can be very comfortable and loving. And allows you to touch your partner easily. If one partner places their leg over the other it will help to bind you together. The spoons position with the man lying behind, is often considered a good way of stimulating the G-spot. If you are feeling exhausted the T-position is helpful: you lie over your partner who lies on his side. Here you control the movement by gently rocking. Above all ensure you are warm, and comfortable.

change location
If you are very much a bedroom couple, consider changing the location: from the bedroom to the bathroom for instance (lit by candles, a warm bubble bath . . .). Even making love on the floor can generate different sensations.

change the timing
Think about the timing of sex: rather than the usual nighttime routine, have an early morning shower and snuggle back into bed with each other. Switch off the TV and go to bed instead!

using sex aids
Sex aids can be fun if you both want to try. A vibrator is the most common sex toy available and you can both try using it to stimulate different parts of the body. Sex aids may not dramatically change your sex life but may help to enhance it or introduce a different

element of excitement.

Remember: *it is your right to seek a healthy, fulfilling sex life and that having a fulfilling intimate life can reflect on the rest of your life in a very positive way. It is also your right to seek help when things go wrong.*

The last word ... why sex is good for you
Dr David Weeks, the head of Old Age Psychology at the Royal Edinburgh Hospital, has spent the past 11 years studying a group of 3,500 people in the UK and America who are considered to be 'super young'. These are people who look, act and often feel far younger than their chronological age. One of his key findings is that the people identified as super young tended to have sex more often – there is, he reports 'lots of great sex in the context of mature, mutually shared erotic unions.'

He says in his book, *Superyoung – the proven way to stay young forever*, Coronet Books, £6.99, that 'in all my years as a clinical psychologist I've never encountered a group of men or women in which there was such a healthy, robust romantic life – and I see many normal, well-adjusted people in my research. By any standard the super young have a remarkably well-developed ability to communicate with their partners and to empathise with one another with great delight which accounts for the greater stability and rich rewards of their relationship.'

Improving the quality of your sex life, advises Dr Weeks, can help make you look between four and seven years younger. He has found that a good sex life can reduce stress and lead to greater contentment.

With an orgasm the body feels good – sex releases a group of substances in the brain, among them beta endorphins, natural painkillers which also alleviate anxiety. Sex also triggers the release of human growth hormone which acts, through another group of peptide hormone substances, to reduce fatty tissues and increase lean muscle in various parts of the body 'giving a more youthful appearance.' Dr Weeks's study also found that sex stimulates the immune system – perhaps by as much as 20%.

During orgasm women produce oxytocin which acts upon the emotional centre of the brain. It plays a part in the nurturing, maternal behaviour – and, says Dr Weeks, 'a lover who regularly stimulates his mate's oxytocin will be rewarded with warmer feelings of affection.' This intense mutual pleasure increases bonding. 'Ongoing sexual frustration probably has an equal and opposite effect: most marriages that crack up are preceded by a decline in the rate of female orgasm.'

Useful further reading

Viagra – A Guide to the Phenomenal Potency–promoting Drug by Dr Susan C. Vaughan, Thorsons, £6.99

Beat The Menopause Without HRT by Maryon Stewart, Headline, £12.99

The Phyto Factor by Maryon Stewart, Vermilion, £8.99

Human Sexuality by Masters and Johnson, Addison Wesley Longman, £24.99

The Virility Solution by Steven Lamm MD, Smallwood Publishing, £19.99

Vitamins and Minerals, An Illustrated Guide by Karen Sullivan, Element, £12.95

Encyclopedia of Complementary Medicine by Anne Woodham and Dr David Peters, Dorling Kindersley, £29.95

Regaining Potency, the answer to male impotence by Oliver Gillie, Self -Help Direct, £10.95

Sex – How To Make It Better for Both of You by Dr Martin Cole and Professor Windy Dryden, Vermilion, £8.99

The Relate Guide to Sex in Loving Relationships by Sarah Litvinoff, Vermilion, £9.99

A Woman's Guide to Loving Sex by Tricia Barnes and Lee Rodwell, Boxtree, £12.99

Self-Help Direct Publishing

Self-Help Direct Publishing was created by two journalists, Oliver Gillie and Michael Crozier, in 1995 to bring important and useful information direct to the public. It aims to provide people with vital facts about health and other matters, so that they may make crucial decisions for themselves. We aim to report on the latest medical advances, drugs and treatments for a variety of conditions which may be hard for those not in the medical profession to learn about.

Books in print:
Regaining Potency: The answer to male impotence by Oliver Gillie
Escape From Pain by Oliver Gillie
Hair Loss: The Answers by Susan Aldridge
You and Your Prostate by Lee Rodwell

About the authors:
◆ **Oliver Gillie** is a leading medical journalist and author. He was medical correspondent of *The Sunday Times* for 15 years and medical editor of *The Independent* for four years. He has a BSc and PhD degrees from Edinburgh University and worked for several years at the National Institute for Medical Research, Mill Hill.

◆ **Susan Aldridge** has a PHD in chemistry and an MSc in biotechnology. Before taking up journalism, she worked for several years as a chemist for the Medical Research Council. Since 1988, she has worked as a freelance journalist and author. She has written three books on genetics and biochemistry.

◆ **Lee Rodwell** is Health Editor of the popular weekly magazine *Take A Break*. Before becoming a full-time freelance health writer, she was a staff journalist on several national newspapers. She has written many books on health and lifestyle issues and her articles have appeared in magazines and newspapers around the world.

◆ **Catherine Kalamis,** neé Catherine Steven, is a former Fleet Street staff reporter and a highly-experienced health writer, journalist and author. She has written three other books on health issues. In 1998 she won the news category of the Medical Journalists Association annual awards and the regional prize of the Rosemary Goodchild/Guild of Health Writers award. She writes regularly for national newspapers and has a weekly health column in the *Guernsey Evening Press*.

Self-Help Direct Publishing, PO Box 9035, London N12 8ED